THE COMPLETE
ILLUSTRATED
GUIDE TO
AYURVEDA

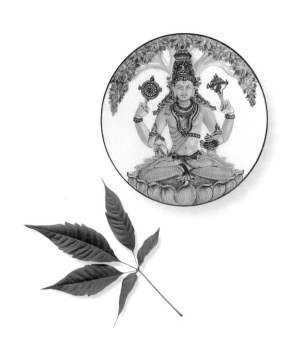

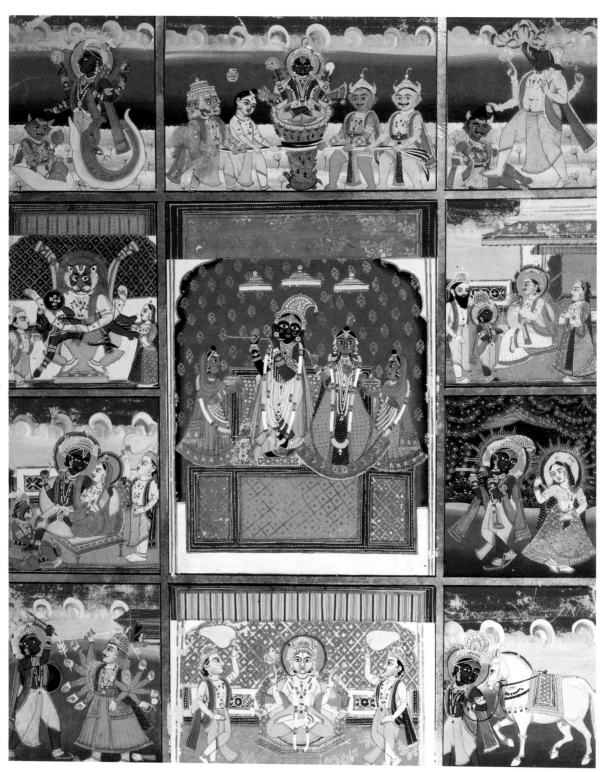

Vishnu surrounded by his ten avatars,
or incarnations.

THE COMPLETE
ILLUSTRATED
GUIDE TO
AYURVEDA

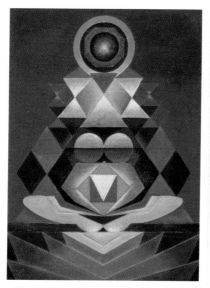

The Ancient Indian
Healing Tradition

GOPI WARRIER AND
DEEPIKA GUNAWANT M.D.

ELEMENT

Shaftesbury, Dorset • Rockport, Massachusetts • Melbourne, Victoria

Designed and created with the Bridgewater Book Company
ELEMENT BOOKS LIMITED
Editorial Director: JULIA McCUTCHEN
Managing Editor: CARO NESS
Production Director: ROGER LANE
Senior Production Controller: SARAH GOLDEN

THE BRIDGEWATER BOOK COMPANY
Art Director: KEVIN KNIGHT
Designer: JANE LANAWAY
Managing Editor: ANNE TOWNLEY
Editor: JULIE WHITAKER
Page make-up: CHRIS LANAWAY
Picture research: VANESSA FLETCHER
Three-dimensional models: MARK JAMIESON
Studio photography: GUY RYECART, IAN PARSONS
Illustrators: LORRAINE HARRISON,
SARAH YOUNG
Computer artwork: JOHN CHRISTOPHER

Printed and bound in
Great Britain by Butler and Tanner, Frome

Acknowledgments

The publishers wish to thank the following for the use of pictures:
Sculpture of Lakshmi, Painting of Cosmic Man by G. Santosh,
and Painting of Oracle by Phung from G. Warrier's collection

Bridgeman Art Library: 2, 6T, 27R, 30, 31B, 61R 66, 97, 142.
et archive: 12T, 141, 170, 171. *The Image Bank*: 6B, 96, 113.
Images Colour Library: 81. *NASA*: 33, 34TL, 34B, 35BR, 172B&T,
173TM. *Rex Features*: 72,161. *Science Photo Library*: 12R, 13L, 39,
48, 57T, 57B, 58, 59TL, 59TR, 59B, 78T, 114, 115, 118L, 118B,
130, 133, 153, 158. *Paul Watts Photography*: 94, 98T, 99L.
Zefa: 7, 26/27, 31T, 73, 99R.

Special thanks go to
Tom Aitken, Tony Bannister, Janine Bennett, Glyn Bridgewater,
Ian Clegg, Viv Croot, Steve Daines, Gail Downey, Ray Goldstein,
Mary Harley, Paul Harley, Kevin Knight, Kay Macmullan,
Norma McLean, Jan O'Boyle, Jerry Phillips,
Paul Spruce, Ian Whitelaw, Krya Wilkie
for help with photography

E O Culverwell, Fogden's Ltd, Shoe Gallery, Bright Ideas, Lewes
Volunteer Bureau, all in Lewes, East Sussex
for help with properties

Authors' Acknowledgments

Lord Ghanapathi Temple and Trustee Mr. Ratnasingam
for photographs of deities. Kamla Jassal for secretarial, nursing
support, and all else. Dr. Krishnakumar of Arya Vaidya Pharmacy
for photographs. Dr. Warrier and Dr. Balachandran of Kottakkal
Arya Vaidya Sala. Chemexcil, India for photographs of herbs.
Gretl, Tyasa, Gillian Torpy, Ruth, Jonathan, Yusuf, Bina, and
Kiri for agreeing to be photographed. Dr. Harsha Thakrar for
agreeing to be photographed. Mr. K. V. Radhakrishnan and
Natesans Galleries for photographs of sculptures. Dr. Mahadevan
for pictures of surgical instruments. Saunder Narayan for translation
from Tamil. Dr. Shastri for phonetic pronunciation
of Sanskrit words. David McAlpine for photographs and the
connection to Michael Mann. Michael Mann Chairman of
Element Books for asking us to write this book. Amy Corzine for
secretarial assistance. Sarah, Lady Morritt for photographs of
paintings. Pallavi, Deepika's daughter. Satish, Deepika's husband.
Shrikala Warrier for Sanskrit calligraphy.

The Ayurvedic theory of creation (*see* pages 32–33) was introduced
by the author at the annual lecture to the National Hindu Students
Federation at the University of Birmingham entitled "New Cosmic
Direction – The creation, preservation and the destruction of the
Universe." The full text of the talk is available © Gopi Warrier.

Dedication

OM
*To Lord Ganapathy, the remover of all obstacles
To Sri Lakshmi, the Goddess of Good Fortune
To Lord Dakshninamoorthy, the great healer and Guru
and to Lord Dhanwantari, the divine physician
as they appear at the churning of the ocean*

Contents

Introduction

AYURVEDA has now become fashionable in the West. Film stars, politicians, and New Age seekers from California to Camden Town, London seek information about Ayurvedic massage and therapy and the best practitioners.

Ayurveda is the oldest complete medical system in the world. Its recorded origins go back about 3,500–4,000 years to the Vedic civilization of India. Ayurveda is part of the *Vedas*, the classical religious texts of Hinduism. References to Ayurveda are found in the *Atharva Veda*, the fourth *Veda*, which deals with herbs, healing, and mantras to cure illness and combat poisons. It has, since then, been the most important medical system of India with effective cures for the most common and chronic ailments of humankind.

Ayurveda is a complete medical system because it has wide-ranging, clearly defined methods of treatment for a variety of ailments and conditions affecting all systems and organs of the body including:

* Musculoskeletal system
* Genitourinary system
* Digestive system
* Circulatory system
* Respiratory system
* Skin and subcutaneous tissue
* Ear, nose, and throat
* Blood-related conditions

Ayurvedic treatment consists mainly of:

* Diagnosis by pulse and clinical examination
* Treatment of the whole body system by balancing the doshas or constituents of the system, i.e., vata, pitta, and kapha
* Detoxification by panchakarma
* Herbal medicines
* Massage

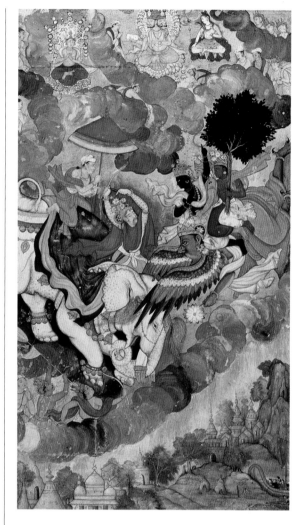

BELOW *The Ayurvedic system of medicine has become popular with people all over the world.*

ABOVE *The Hindu god Krishna, on the fabulous bird Garuda, overcomes Indra seated on his elephant.*

The purpose of this book is to act as a general guide to individuals and practitioners who want to understand their own body system better according to the philosophy of Ayurveda and to go on to a higher level of academic training if they wish to pursue it as a career.

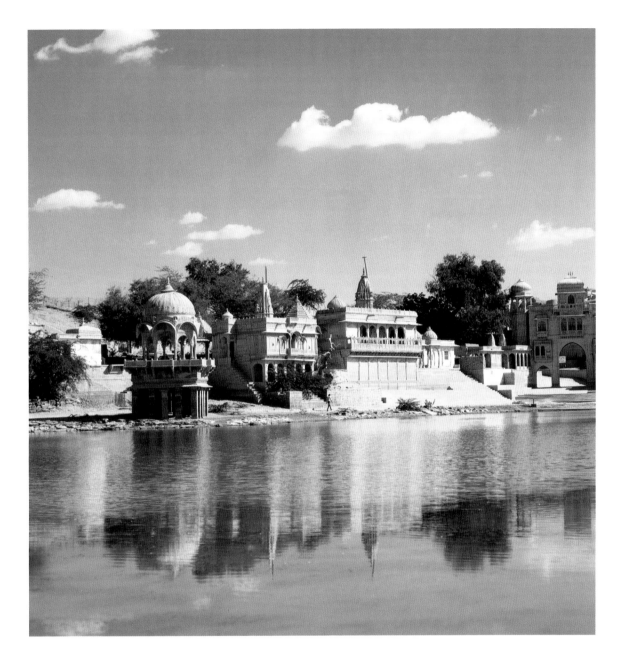

It is not intended as a guide for treatment of other people as this requires a rigorous and long period of training of at least five years, in a proper university environment, where the fundamentals including anatomy, physiology, botany, and the pharmacopoeia of Ayurveda are clearly understood, not to mention the practical training involved.

In the current world scenario Western countries use economic, political, and media power to create barriers to the entry of herbal products from devel-

ABOVE *Many Hindu temples, like this beautiful building in Jaisalmer, Rajasthan, in northwest India, are built beside purifying lakes and in beautiful natural surroundings.*

oping countries, thus depriving them of income and the Western public of a potential cure for their illnesses. The power of Ayurveda can be correctly reinvoked only for the benefit of humanity as a whole and for universal physical and spiritual revival regardless of wealth, creed, or nationality.

How to Use this Book

As Ayurvedic medicine increases in popularity in the West, and ever more people turn to its wisdom and methods in their search for spiritual well-being and physical health, there is a need for a book such as this one. Chapter by chapter, *The Complete Illustrated Guide to Ayurveda* provides an overview of this ancient science, its history, its philosophy, its methods and medicines, in order to help the individual understand his or her own body system better and to improve their quality of life.

This book is not intended as a manual for the would-be practitioner of Ayurvedic healing, for the necessary period of training is a minimum of five years' academic study. The practice of Ayurveda requires a thorough grounding in a wide range of medical disciplines, including anatomy and physiology, and the physician must have a deep understanding of the history and theory behind the Ayurvedic pharmacopoeia. Anyone wishing to pursue Ayurveda as a career should go on to a higher level of academic training, and it is to be hoped that this book will encourage many to do so.

The first chapter of the book introduces the basic tenets of Ayurveda, and the claims, aims, and methods of this ancient art of healing.

The second chapter provides an overview of the history of this rich body of knowledge, and the fundamental myths and theories of Ayurveda.

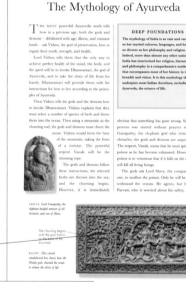

The history and myths of Ayurveda are illustrated with full color images of Indian artifacts, including gods and mythical scenes.

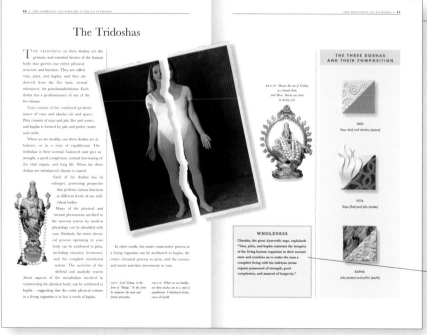

The third chapter of the book examines the principles and categories that are fundamental to the Ayurvedic view of the human physical and mental condition. The key terms and concepts, such as the tridoshas (which must be brought into balance if good health is to be achieved) are fully explained, using simple examples and clear images. The different types of people, and the kinds of illness from which they tend to suffer, are discussed in detail.

Boxed features highlight quotations from the ancient masters of Ayurveda.

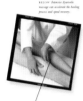

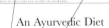

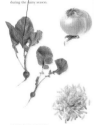

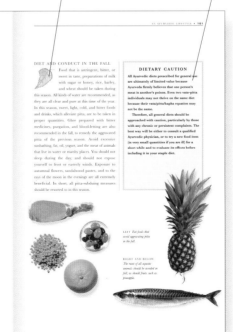

Ayurveda and Modern Medicine Working Together

In the fourth chapter, the role of Ayurveda in the modern world, both in India and in the West, is examined – the training, the medicines, and the scientific evidence of their benefits.

Individual case studies show the proven benefits of the Ayurvedic method.

Complementary uses of Western and Ayurvedic medical techniques are illustrated.

The fifth chapter provides detailed advice on how to adapt our lives to the Ayurvedic way, through daily and seasonal routines that can help us to keep our bodies in harmonious balance and avoid illness. Diet, work, hygiene, and meditation are all discussed.

Graphic images help to convey the key concepts of Ayurveda.

Specific routines are given for each season of the year.

Recurring symbols enable the reader to understand the underlying theory.

Key aspects of Ayurveda are highlighted in special boxes.

An Ayurvedic Diet

The sixth and seventh chapters outline the principal ways of diagnosing, classifying, and treating diseases through the application of Ayurvedic philosophy and methods. Treatments include a wide range of techniques, from external medicine and surgery, to astrology and rejuvenation.

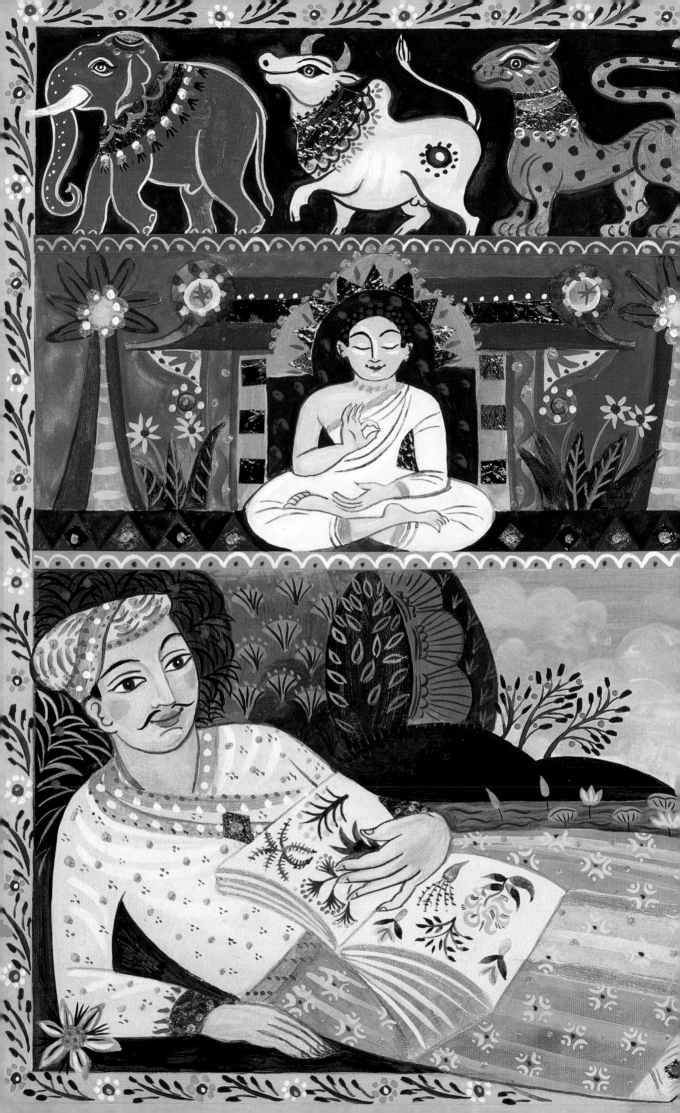

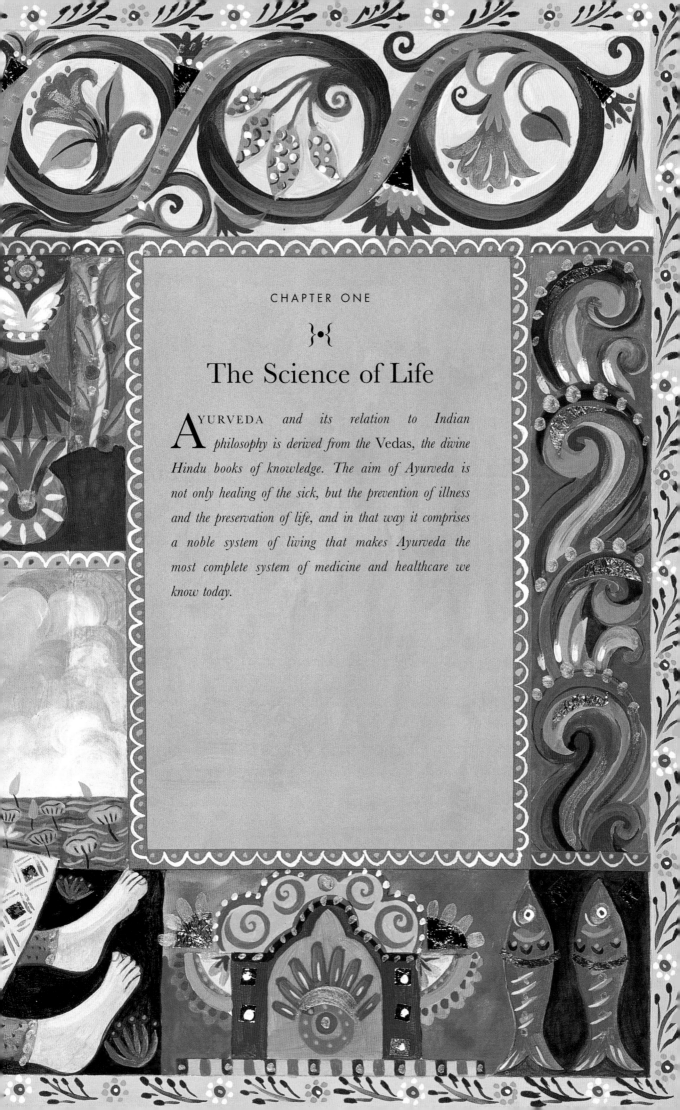

}•{

The Science of Life

AYURVEDA *and its relation to Indian philosophy is derived from the* Vedas, *the divine Hindu books of knowledge. The aim of Ayurveda is not only healing of the sick, but the prevention of illness and the preservation of life, and in that way it comprises a noble system of living that makes Ayurveda the most complete system of medicine and healthcare we know today.*

What is Ayurveda?

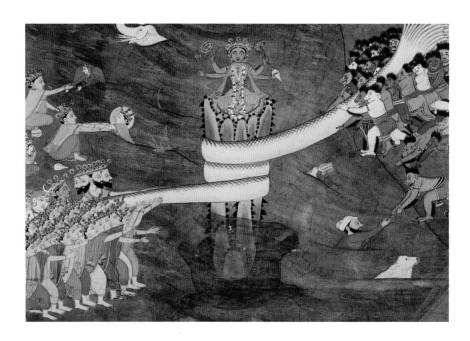

AYURVEDA is a Sanskrit word derived from two roots, "Ayus" and "vid," meaning life and knowledge respectively. Ayus, or life, represents a combination of the body, the sense organs, the mind, and the soul. The *Vedas* are ancient Hindu books of knowledge that are said to have been divinely revealed to the sages of India many thousands of years ago. They contain within them the knowledge, the rhythm, and the structure of the universe and the secrets of sickness and health. There are four *Vedas*, *Rig Veda*, *Sama Veda*, *Yajur Veda*, and *Atharva Veda*. Ayurveda is part of this fourth *Veda*, which includes detailed dissertations upon the treatment of the sick using mantras, herbs, and potions. Ayurveda is a combination of science and philosophy, which details the many physical,

ABOVE *In Hindu mythology the gods churn the cosmic ocean to obtain ambrosia, or the elixir of life.*

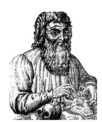

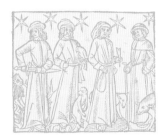

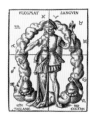

The *Rig Veda*, containing hymns to the gods, is the first of four *Vedas*, the divinely revealed Indian books of wisdom.

The fourth *Veda* – the *Atharva Veda* – is written, containing the ancient wisdom about sickness and healing upon which Ayurvedic treatment is founded.

Hippocrates, an eminent Greek physician and teacher, writes about methods of healing, and identifies some of the effects of environment on health.

Galen, another Greek physician and medical teacher, carries out experiments and makes important discoveries about nerves and the muscles that control breathing. He develops

complex ideas about the circulatory and nervous systems, and extends Hippocrates' theory that our bodies are governed by the four humors – blood, phlegm, black and yellow bile.

1500 BCE   800 BCE   400 BCE   AD 150

mental, emotional, and spiritual components necessary for holistic health. The sophistication of this system is apparent in the most famous of all ancient Ayurvedic texts, the *Charaka Samhita*.

This important document of internal medicine, which was written more than 2,000 years before the microscope was invented, explains how the body is made up of cells, and it lists 20 different microscopic organisms that may cause disease. Another of the texts, the *Sushruta Samhita*, explains surgical methods, surgical equipment, suturing, and the importance of hygiene during and after an operation. Detailed medical information is combined with spiritual and philosophical advice on how to live a healthy and purposeful life. According to Vedic philosophy human lives will be filled with purpose when they strive to fulfill their full potential, but that cannot be achieved without health on a basic level. All modern Ayurvedic practitioners work in accordance with traditional beliefs and practices.

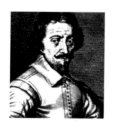

ABOVE *One of the key works of Indian medicine, the* Charaka Samhita, *explained more than 2,000 years ago that the body is composed of cells.*

SANSKRIT FOR AYUS
Ayus means life.

SANSKRIT FOR VID
Vid means science. Ayus and vid together make Ayurveda, the science of life.

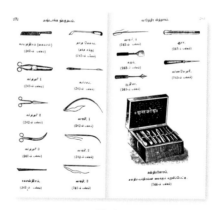

ABOVE *The* Sushruta Samhita *is the most important text on surgery in ancient India.*

The theory of four humors, which create sanguine, phlegmatic, melancholic, and choleric emotions, continues to hold sway in Europe.

1543

The Flemish physician Andreas Vesalius draws the first accurate pictures of the human anatomy, based on studies of corpses.

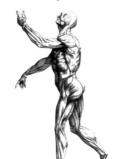

1590

Dutchman Zacharias Janssen (above) invents the microscope, enabling the study of cells and leading to the discovery of bacteria.

Scottish bacteriologist Alexander Fleming realizes that mold in a plate is killing off bacteria. He has discovered penicillin, the first antibiotic.

By injecting cowpox, the English physician Edward Jenner successfully protects a boy against smallpox – the first vaccination.

1796

1928

What is Ayurvedic Medicine?

AYURVEDIC medicine is the traditional, all-embracing national system of medicine practiced in India and Sri Lanka. Ayurveda is a comprehensive system of healthcare and its many elements work together prescribing a way of life, rather than a treatment for specific illnesses. Some of the elements of Ayurvedic medicine include:

❖ Detoxification by panchakarma

❖ Diet

❖ Yoga

❖ Herbal medication

❖ Meditation and prayer

The basic Ayurvedic belief is that everything within the universe, including ourselves, is composed of five elements called panchamahabhutas and tridoshas. By correcting the balance of the tridoshas within ourselves and in relation to the world around us, we will promote health on all levels.

Ayurvedic treatment is tailored to the individual. There is no one treatment that works for an ailment in every person. The combination of the doshas that make up one person might lead to optimum health for them. In another person, that balance of doshas may cause illness. In Ayurvedic medicine every person must be treated individually. The skill of the practitioner lies in assessing each individual's constitution (*see* The Prakrti, page 66), diagnosing the causes of any imbalance, identifying the constitutional type and where the balance of doshas lie, and deciding upon the best possible treatment.

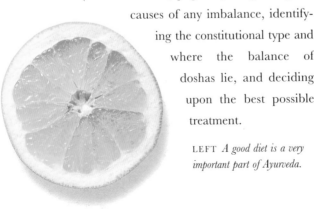

LEFT *A good diet is a very important part of Ayurveda.*

THE EIGHT BRANCHES

There are eight branches of Ayurveda, which are practically integrated on every level. They include detailed treatises on:

❖ Surgery

❖ Medicine

❖ Gynecology

❖ Pediatrics

❖ Toxicology

❖ Otorhinolaryngology (ears, nose, and throat)

❖ Rejuvenation

❖ Virilification therapy

LEFT *Undivided India, known as "sacred land."*

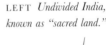

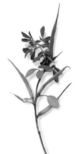

ABOVE *Ayurvedic medicine contains many herbal ingredients.*

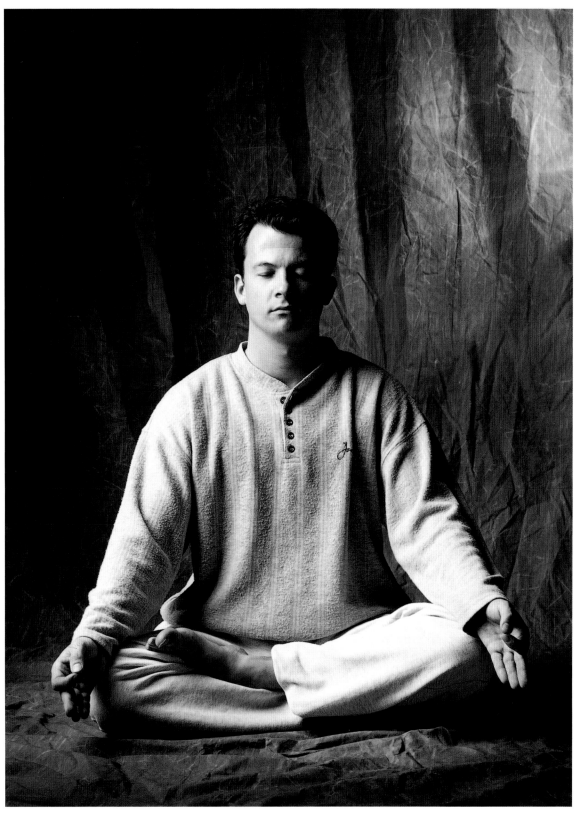

ABOVE *Meditation is part
of Ayurvedic prayer.*

The Aim of Ayurveda

AYURVEDA is an excellent guide for health, and living in a good and moral way. Like many holistic therapies, the emphasis is on the mind, body, and spirit – and in Ayurveda that spirituality is intrinsic to good health and a noble way of life. It aims not only to cure diseases but also to create health and well-being.

Ayurvedic theory is based on the individual constitution of a person, according to which he or she is susceptible to certain illnesses. Ayurveda considers the influence of psychosomatic factors in most of the diseases and the imbalance of the basic constitutional factors that is responsible for causing an illness.

Treatment is aimed at restoring the disturbed mechanism. The basic constitutional factors are the three doshas – vata, pitta, and kapha – and restoration of their dynamic balance regulates the life cycle and controls the entire body, so restoring health.

PREVENTION IS BETTER THAN CURE

The aim of Ayurveda is not only healing the sick, but the prevention of illness and preservation of life. The Ayurvedic theory of creation discusses factors that are interlinked, including:

✤ The body
✤ The mind
✤ The soul or the consciousness
✤ The panchamahabhutas (the five elements)

These factors are complementary to each other, and are equally important in every person. Ayurveda is a "holistic" system of medicine, which means that it treats the person as a whole, not as a group of individual parts. Ayurveda is aimed at treating the mind, body, and spirit.

RIGHT *The emphasis of the Ayurvedic method of healing is on restoring balance, and therefore health, to the mind, body, and spirit.*

The physical body is only one of four factors that make up the whole individual.

The restoration and maintenance of balance is the key to health and well-being.

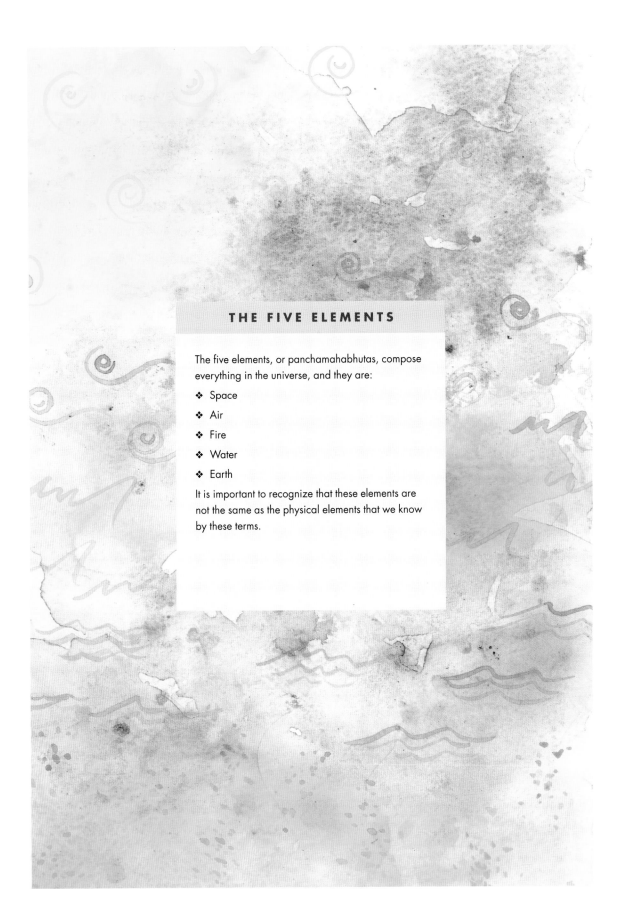

THE FIVE ELEMENTS

The five elements, or panchamahabhutas, compose everything in the universe, and they are:

❖ Space

❖ Air

❖ Fire

❖ Water

❖ Earth

It is important to recognize that these elements are not the same as the physical elements that we know by these terms.

How Does it Work?

AYURVEDIC medicine is based on the principle that every individual person has a unique constitution that is related to energies within the body. A good, balanced constitution is the best defense against illness. If your body is functioning at optimum level, there is no way for ill health to gain a stronghold. However, a poorly balanced constitution makes one susceptible to illness – both physical and mental. Ayurveda aims to prevent the development of disease by working with the constitution of the individual. Our constitutions are determined by the balance of three vital energies in the body, known as the three doshas, or tridoshas. The three doshas are known by their Sanskrit names of vata, pitta, and kapha. Each individual constitution is controlled by all three doshas to different degrees, but we usually have one, or possibly two, dominant doshas. A practitioner will assess your constitution and determine the prakrti to which you belong.

Doshas not only determine the characteristics of our constitutions, and the type of illnesses to which we are most likely to succumb, they also determine the features that make us unique – like the color of our hair, our body shape, our cravings for food, and what foods we should eat. Every single aspect of our lives is affected by the doshas.

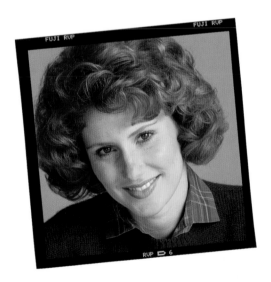

| YOUR PRAKRTI |
You may be classed as one of the following types:

* vata   * vata–pitta
* pitta   * pitta–kapha
* kapha   * vata–kapha

Good health reigns when all three doshas work in balance. Each one has its role to play in the body. For example, vata produces movement and relates mainly to the nervous system and the body's energy. Pitta is fire; it relates to the metabolism, digestion, enzymes, acid, and bile. Kapha is related to water in the mucous membranes, phlegm, moisture, fat, and lymphatics. The balance of the three doshas depends on a variety of factors, in particular correct diet and exercise, good digestion, healthy elimination of body wastes, and balanced emotional and spiritual health.

Each constitution is determined by the state of the parental doshas at the time of conception. Each individual is born with a typical prakrti, a mixture of doshas unique to him or her. This is your constitution and it remains with you for life. But, as we travel through life, diet, environment, stress, trauma, and injury cause the doshas to become imbalanced, a state known as the "vikrti" state. When levels of imbalance are excessively high or low, ill health can result. Ayurvedic practitioners work to restore each individual to the best balance possible within their prakrti.

Constitutions are inborn and cannot be changed. Ayurvedic philosophy understands and accepts the differences between individuals, and everyone's uniqueness. The science of Ayurveda helps us to

LEFT *Doshas determine the uniqueness of our features, such as the color of eyes and hair, and body shape.*

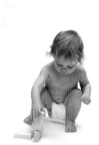

RIGHT *Our constitutions and prakrti are determined even in the womb of the mother.*

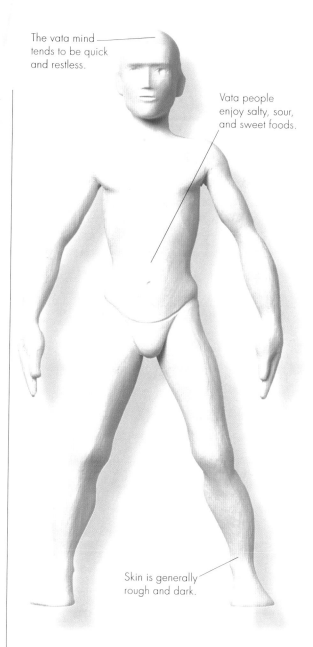

SANSKRIT FOR VATA

The vata mind tends to be quick and restless.

Vata people enjoy salty, sour, and sweet foods.

Skin is generally rough and dark.

ABOVE *The vata body type tends to be thin, with light bone structure.*

understand our own constitutions and to live in a way that emphasizes their positive aspects – which is not always easy.

In Ayurveda, all ill health is related to disturbances in these three doshas. Doshic imbalances affect other factors at work in the body, and lead to imbalances that cause disease. These other factors include the five elements (panchamahabhutas), the ten pairs of qualities of the tridoshas, agni, the three malas, and the seven tissues (sapha dhathus). These factors will be discussed in more detail in Chapter Three: The Principles of Ayurveda, and in Chapter Five: An Ayurvedic Lifestyle.

The body and the mind can be the home of disease as easily as of well-being. Well-being is achieved through the balance of the biological units, and disease is an imbalance of the units. The objective of Ayurveda is to re-establish equilibrium when we are ill, and to maintain that equilibrium in order to keep us healthy.

HARMONY

Good health, according to Ayurvedic philosophy, is a state of balance between the mind, body, spirit, and environment. This balance, or harmony, is achieved through diet, yoga, lifestyle, and meditation.

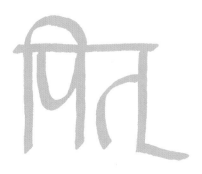

SANSKRIT FOR PITTA

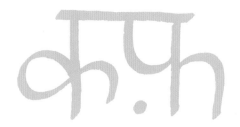

SANSKRIT FOR KAPHA

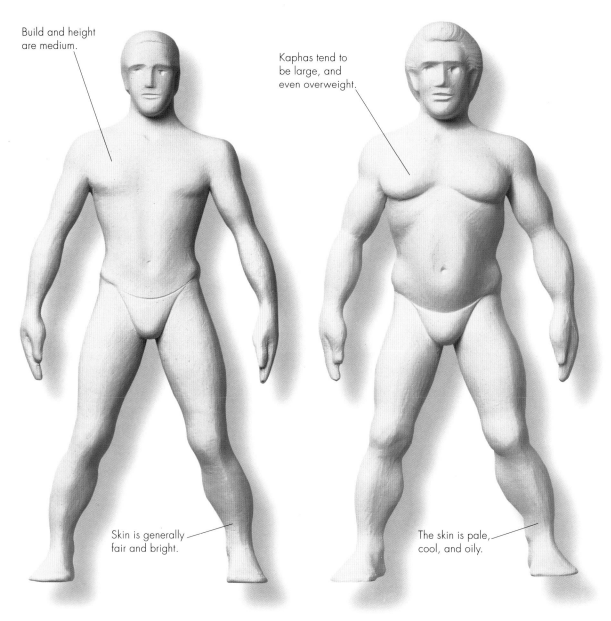

Build and height
are medium.

Kaphas tend to
be large, and
even overweight.

Skin is generally
fair and bright.

The skin is pale,
cool, and oily.

ABOVE *The pitta body type tends*
to be of medium build, with fair,
freckled skin, and reddish hair.

ABOVE *The kapha body type is*
large-framed and slightly overweight.

The Three Doshas

VATA

❖ Vatas' elements are air and space.

❖ Air is the dominant element with qualities of light, cold, dry, rough, subtle, mobile, clear, dispersing, erratic, and astringent.

❖ Vata people tend to be thin with dry, rough, and dark skin; large, crooked, or protruding teeth; a small thin mouth; and dull, dark eyes.

❖ Vatas speak quickly, sleep little, and their sleep is often interrupted. They are very active and have a quick, restless mind. They are good at

ABOVE *Air is the dominant element in the vata person.*

remembering recent events, but have a poor long-term memory. They are changeable in their beliefs.

❖ They are often frightened and anxious, and can have an unpredictable temper.

❖ Vatas eat little. They like sweet, sour, and salty foods and are moderately thirsty. They are often constipated.

❖ Vata people tend to be emotionally insecure.

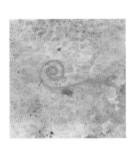

AIR

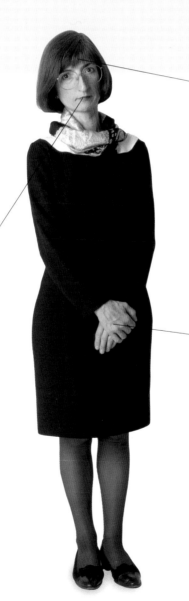

Vatas have poor long-term memory.

Vatas speak quickly, and have an active and restless mind.

Vata people often have dry skin.

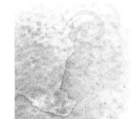

SPACE

BELOW *Vatas are fond of sweet foods.*

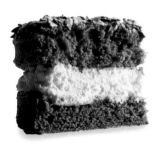

LEFT *The vata person tends to be thin, highly active, and mentally restless. Emotionally, they are often frightened and insecure.*

PITTA

❖ Pittas' elements are fire and water.

❖ Pitta qualities are light, hot, oily, sharp, liquid, sour, and pungent.

❖ Pittas are usually of medium height and build, with soft, fair skin; light brown or reddish hair; small yellowish teeth; a medium-sized mouth; and penetrating green, gray, or yellowish eyes.

❖ Pittas speak clearly, but often sharply. They enjoy light but uninterrupted sleep.

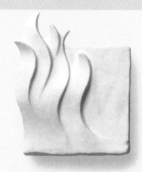

ABOVE *Fire is the dominant element in the pitta person.*

❖ Pittas are intelligent, but often aggressively so, have a good clear memory, and can be fanatic in their beliefs. Pittas tend to be jealous, aggressive, and easily irritated.

❖ Pittas love to eat and they eat a lot; they like sweet, bitter, and sharp-tasting foods; and have an unquenchable thirst.

❖ Bowel movements are regular, with soft, loose stools.

❖ Pittas tend to be emotionally intense.

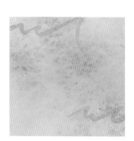

FIRE

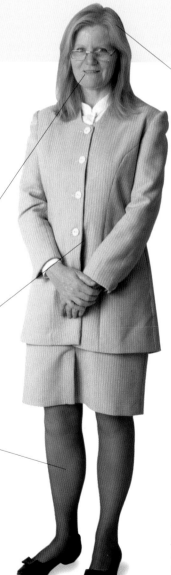

Pittas usually have soft, fair hair.

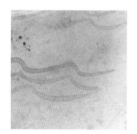

WATER

Many pittas have a freckled and bright skin.

They have a strong digestion and like sharp-tasting, sweet, and bitter foods.

Pitta types tend to be of medium build.

RIGHT *Of medium build, and with fair skin and fair or reddish hair, the pitta person tends to be intelligent with a good memory.*

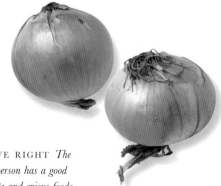

ABOVE RIGHT *The pitta person has a good appetite and enjoys foods with strong flavors.*

KAPHA

❖ Kaphas' elements are water and earth.

❖ Kapha qualities are heavy, cold, oily, slow, slimy, dense, soft, static, and sweet.

❖ Kaphas are usually large framed and perhaps overweight.

❖ Skin is thick, pale, cool, and oily; hair is thick, wavy, and oily. Mouths tend to be large with full lips, and eyes are big and often beautiful with thick, dark lashes.

❖ Kaphas speak slowly and need a great deal of sleep. They need time

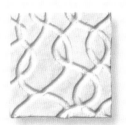

ABOVE *Water is the element that dominates in the kapha person.*

to think things through calmly and rationally.

❖ Kaphas have a long memory but are slow to learn and have poor short-term recall.

❖ Kaphas stick to their beliefs, can be calm and caring but also greedy and possessive.

❖ Kaphas have a slow, steady appetite and enjoy bitter, pungent, and sharp tastes.

❖ Bowel movements are slow.

❖ Kaphas are very loving and emotionally secure.

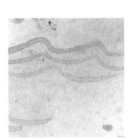

WATER

Kaphas like to think things through rationally.

Skin is thick, cool, and oily.

Kaphas are often of large build.

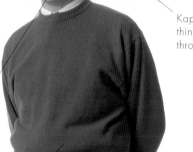

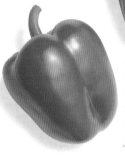

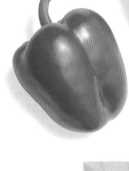

ABOVE LEFT *Sharp and pungent tastes are the kapha person's favorites.*

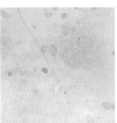

EARTH

RIGHT *With a large frame, the kapha person tends to be slow, caring, and emotionally secure.*

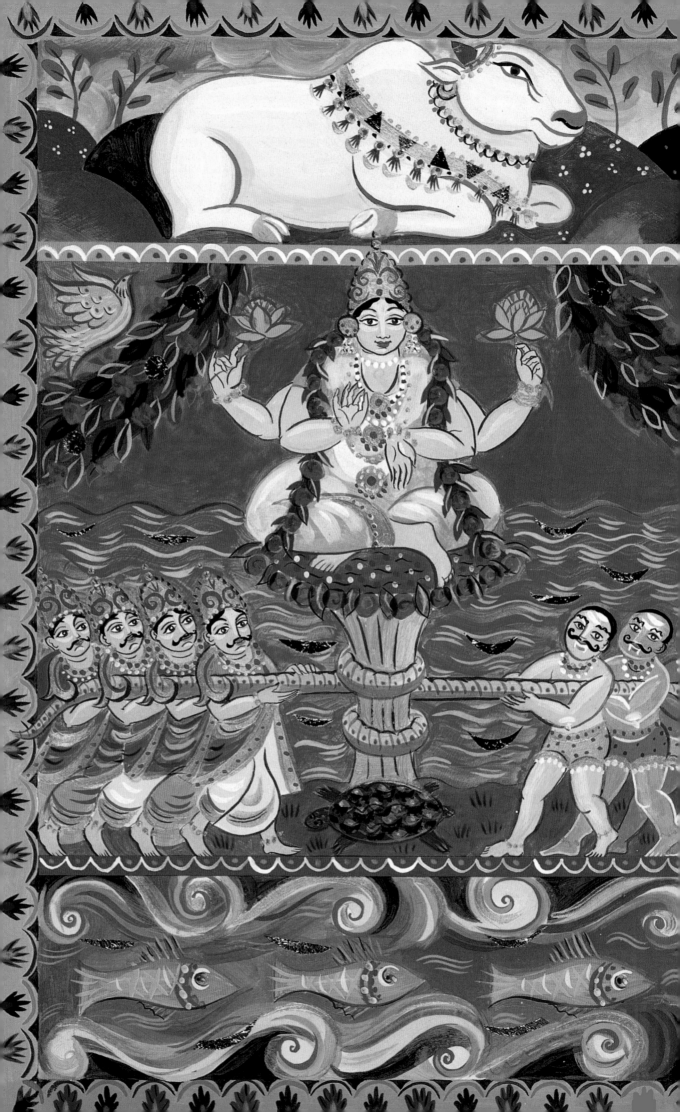

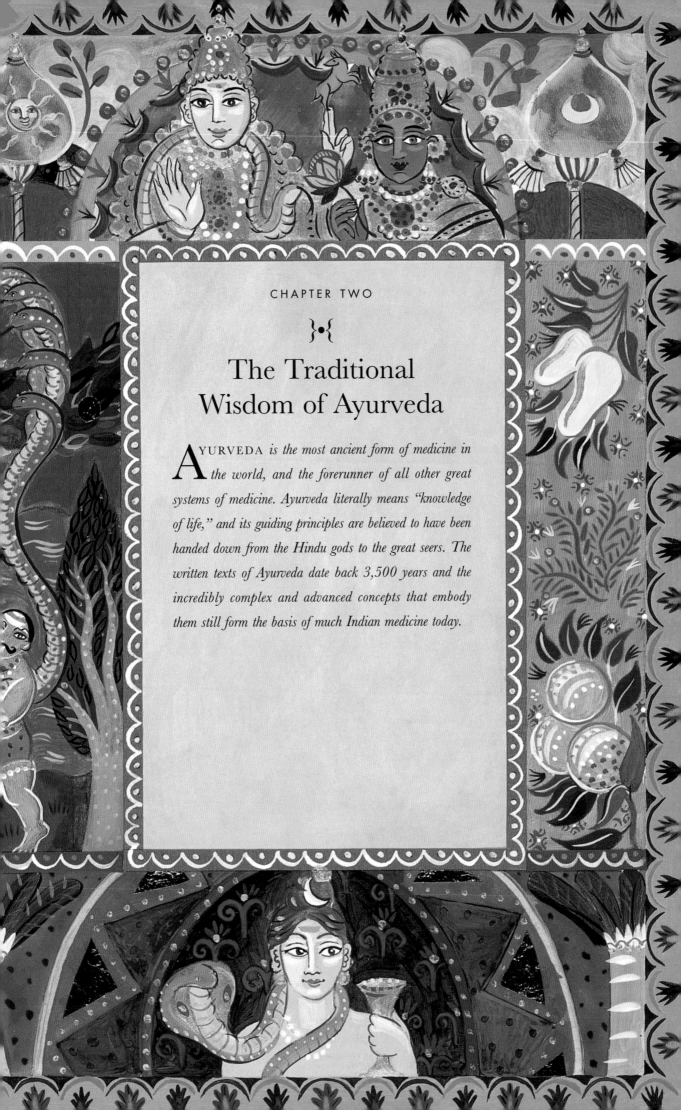

CHAPTER TWO

The Traditional
Wisdom of Ayurveda

A YURVEDA *is the most ancient form of medicine in the world, and the forerunner of all other great systems of medicine. Ayurveda literally means "knowledge of life," and its guiding principles are believed to have been handed down from the Hindu gods to the great seers. The written texts of Ayurveda date back 3,500 years and the incredibly complex and advanced concepts that embody them still form the basis of much Indian medicine today.*

The Meaning of Ayurveda

WE LEARNED in Chapter One that Ayurveda is a Sanskrit word derived from two roots, "Ayus" and "vid," meaning life and knowledge respectively. Ayus, or life, represents a combination of the body, the sense organs, the mind, and the soul. Therefore, broadly speaking, Ayurveda means knowledge concerning the maintenance of life.

Ayurveda aims to prevent illness and to balance the mind, body, and spirit. This doctrine means that people are treated before illness has a chance to manifest itself. An Ayurvedic practitioner will assess and monitor the lifestyle of every patient – including their diet, personal habits, hobbies, relationships, sex life, working and home conditions, spirituality, and every other aspect of daily life – in order to provide advice that will ensure that imbalances do not occur.

Ayurveda is deeply rooted in the mythology of India, and in its religious beliefs. Myth, legend, religion, and daily living are interrelated, and the mantras used in Ayurvedic healing are part of the normal, unconscious routine in many orthodox Indian households.

BELOW RIGHT *An Ayurvedic physician will ask the patient about his or her lifestyle and working patterns.*

RIGHT *Spirituality plays a very important part in the everyday life of India, with daily visits to the temple to pray for guidance and help.*

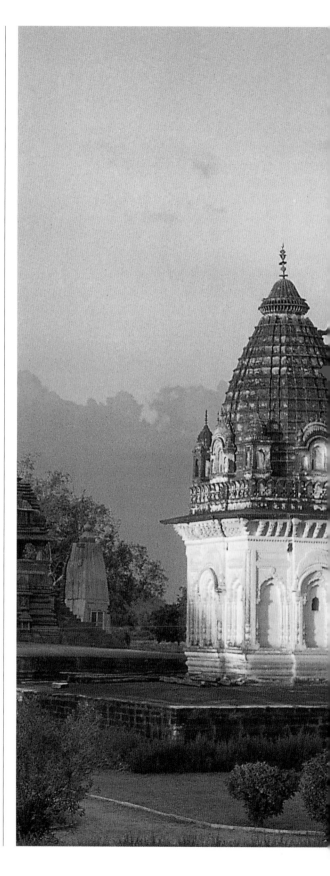

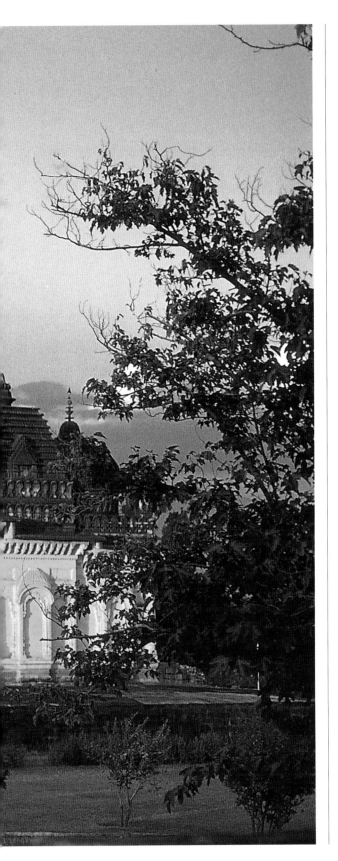

ANCIENT WISDOM

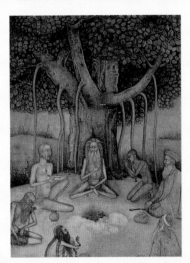

Charaka, the great Ayurvedic sage, wrote, "That is designated as Ayurveda or the Science of Life wherein are laid down the good and the bad of life, the happy and unhappy life, and what is wholesome and what is unwholesome of life, as also the measure of life."

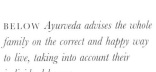

BELOW *Ayurveda advises the whole family on the correct and happy way to live, taking into account their individual karma.*

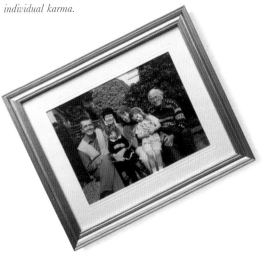

The Mythology of Ayurveda

THE MOST powerful Ayurvedic myth tells how in a previous age, both the gods and demons – debilitated with age, illness, and constant battle – ask Vishnu, the god of preservation, how to regain their youth, strength, and health.

Lord Vishnu tells them that the only way to achieve perfect health of the mind, the body, and the spirit will be to invoke Dhanwantari, the god of Ayurveda, and to take the elixir of life from his hands. Dhanwantari will provide them with his instructions for how to live according to the principles of Ayurveda.

Then Vishnu tells the gods and the demons how to invoke Dhanwantari. Vishnu explains that they must select a number of species of herb and throw them into the ocean. Then using a mountain as the churning rod, the gods and demons must churn the ocean. Vishnu would form the base of the mountain, taking the form of a tortoise. The powerful serpent Vasuki will be the churning rope.

The gods and demons follow these instructions, the selected herbs are thrown into the sea, and the churning begins. However, it is immediately

obvious that something has gone wrong. Since the process was started without prayers to Lord Ganapathy, the elephant god who removes all obstacles, the gods and demons are unprotected. The serpent, Vasuki, warns that he must spit out his poison as he has become exhausted. However, his poison is so venomous that if it falls on the earth, it will kill all living beings.

The gods ask Lord Shiva, the compassionate one, to swallow the poison. Only he will be able to withstand the venom. He agrees, but his wife Parvati, who is worried about his safety, runs to

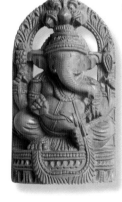

ABOVE *Lord Ganapathy, the elephant-headed remover of all obstacles and son of Shiva.*

The churning begins with the god Vishnu as the base of the mountain.

RIGHT *This carved sandalwood box shows how the Hindu gods churned the ocean to obtain the elixir of life.*

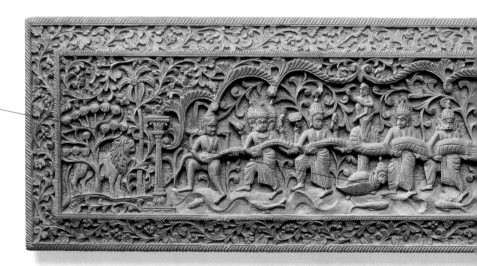

Shiva and squeezes his neck as tightly as she can in order to prevent the poison from flowing down. The poison remains in his throat, but it colors Shiva's neck blue – hence his other name, "Neelakanda," the blue-necked one.

Vishnu realizes why these problems have arisen and he instructs all the assembled gods and demons to pray to Ganapathy. After that they can restart the churning.

As the churning proceeds, gems, beautiful trees, elephants, and Lakshmi, the goddess of wealth, come out of the ocean. Finally, the god Dhanwantari comes out of the ocean bearing the elixir of life in his hands. But before the gods can greet him, the elixir is snatched from his hands by the demons, who run away.

The gods again ask Vishnu to help, and this time he adopts the form of a seductive angel and persuades the demons to close their eyes to eat the elixir. As soon as their eyes are closed, Vishnu takes the elixir and returns it to the gods who consume it quickly to regain their radiance.

The myth illustrates the effort that is required to resuscitate the ecological balance of the earth herself – to protect her resources and biodiversity and to divide them fairly, before demonic beings can grab what should be distributed to all.

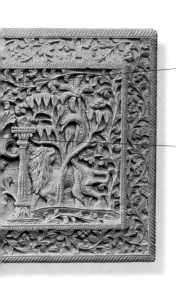

Dhanwantari comes out of the ocean bearing the elixir of life.

The gods churn the sea of milk with Vasuki, the serpent.

THE HINDU PANTHEON

Although many divinities may be worshipped, modern Hindus are generally divided into followers of Vishnu, Shiva, or Shakti.

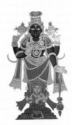

Vishnu is the protector and preserver of the world, and he is worshipped by many faiths in various forms. The worship of this god is called Vaisnavism.

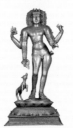

Shiva is Sanskrit for "auspicious one," and is a more remote god than Vishnu. His worship is called Shivaism. He is regarded as both destroyer and restorer.

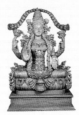

The worship of Shakti is the worship of the mother goddess, either individually as Lakshmi, the goddess of wealth; Kali and Durga, both goddesses of destruction and protection; and Saraswati, the goddess of wisdom and learning. They are also worshipped collectively as Shakti or as Sri Maha Tripurasundari the triple goddesses.

A POWERFUL SAVIOR

It is part of the enduring power of Ayurveda that whenever mankind is threatened with incurable disease, debilitation, and a confrontational frame of mind, Ayurveda emerges from the eternally vibrant "Vedic space" to rejuvenate humanity and the world.

A Brief History of Ayurvedic Texts

IN INDIA there is a saying that wealth earned from medical practice and the legal profession is always contaminated as it comes from the suffering of others. Ayurveda is said to have been handed down divinely, and it must be practiced with compassion and nobility, not greed or egoism.

The main source of Ayurvedic knowledge is the *Vedas,* the divine Hindu books of knowledge. The *Vedas* were revealed by Lord Brahma, the creator of this universe according to Hindu mythology. From him the inspired sages received this knowledge, and then passed it on to others.

The *Vedas* are made up of four texts. The *Rig Veda* is the oldest, with a collection of 1,028 hymns. The *Yajur Veda* and *Sama Veda* are the backbone of Indian religion and philosophy, dating from 3000 BCE. The fourth *Veda* is the *Atharva Veda,* which dates from about 1200 BCE, and this is the main source book for Ayurveda, the Indian system of medicine and treatment.

Further classical Ayurvedic texts were written from 600 BCE to AD 1000. Three great authors compiled the *Brihattraye:* they were Charaka, Sushruta, and Vaghbhatta. Medicine was revealed by Indra to Atreya, which finally led to the Charaka tradition of general medicine.

Surgery was revealed by Indra to Divodasa, the king of Kasi, who was also an incarnation of the divine Dhanwantari. This led to the Sushruta tradition of Ayurvedic surgery. Vaghbhatta wrote his main book *Astanga Samgraha,* summarizing the view of Charaka and Sushruta, and putting forward his own thoughts on the management of diseases.

Over the years, a vast pharmacopoeia was added to this knowledge and the Ayurvedic tradition continued as a vigorous and fast-expanding scientific tradition down into the 16th century. The 20th century has seen scientific trials on many Ayurvedic medicines, proving their safety and efficacy.

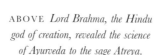

ABOVE *Lord Brahma, the Hindu god of creation, revealed the science of Ayurveda to the sage Atreya.*

BELOW *Holy sage addressing his followers. Ayurvedic knowledge was composed and handed down over centuries.*

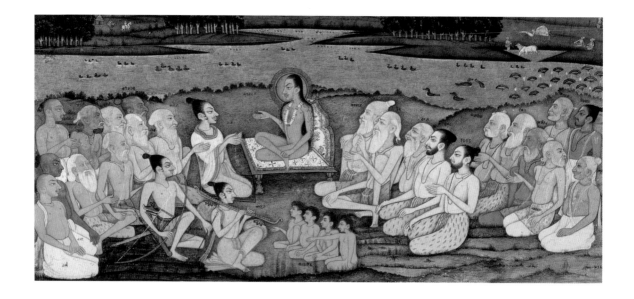

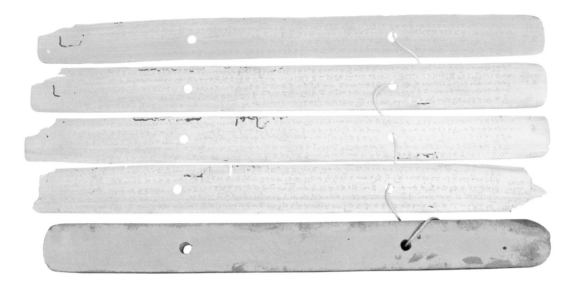

ABOVE *This historical Ayurvedic textbook is written in Sanskrit and made of bamboo wood.*

THE VEDAS

Although it was meant to have been divinely revealed many thousands of years ago, it was sometime between **1500** and **1200** BCE that the *Rig Veda* was actually written down. It is the oldest religious scripture in the world. Three other collections – the *Sama Veda, Yajur Veda,* and *Atharva Veda* – were added later. These were all composed over a period of several centuries and collected in their present form during the first millennium BCE.

MAIN INFLUENCES

There are many philosophies in India, such as Samkhya, Nyaya, Vaisheshika, Vedanta, and others, but the dominant intellectual influences on Ayurveda are those of the Samkhya and the Vaisheshika Indian philosophies. The Samkhya philosophy greatly influenced Indian medicine, particularly through the theory of Yoga.

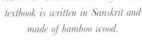

INDRA

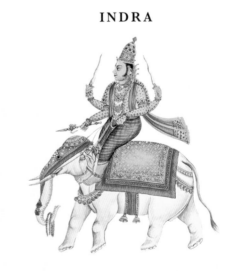

In the Vedic period, Indra was the king of the gods, and lord of the storm, fertility, and war. Indra and the other primary gods of the *Vedas,* named Brahma, Agni, and Varuna, were displaced by newer deities – in particular, Shiva, Vishnu, and Shakti – who have many followers today.

The Ayurvedic Theory of Creation

THE FUNDAMENTAL entities of all life according to Ayurveda are the panchamahabhutas, or the five elements: earth, water, fire, air, and space. From the combination of these elements arise the forces of vata (air and space), pitta (fire and water), and kapha (water and earth). These entities structure the manifested world and the cosmic being (purusha). To the uninitiated individual lost in the veil of illusion (maya) the different aspects of the cosmic being seem like the manifested world. This physical, or illusionary universe, is called prakrti.

The creation that we see is simply the different facets of the cosmic being itself undergoing the process of change according to the ripple created within its own system by the forces of vata, pitta, and kapha.

Individual consciousness corresponds to the dream state of the cosmic being. This cosmic dream state called "Vaiswanara" coincides with the state of humanity living under the illusion of reality – without realizing that we are all part of one giant dream. This kapha state in humanity is represented by the god Brahma who is called the creator. It represents the potential energy of the universe at rest, while its mind refreshes itself through the cleaning crackle of neurons in dreams. Neurologists have already studied this phenomenon in human sleep and call it REM (Rapid Eye Movement).

The sleep of the Cosmic Being is called Brahma niara.

RIGHT *The cosmic being is like a tree with its root above and the branches below.*

According to the author's theory, the "Big Bang" happened when the cosmic brain's "neurons," driven by cosmic kapha forces to hibernate in its cosmic center (brain), exploded like the REMs in sleep, creating the illusion of the universe.

This dream state of the cosmic being represents the earliest forms of life on earth (viral and bacterial), as well as unevolved human beings who are still engrossed with the external world, believing it to be true. But they are simply neural movements of the sleeping cosmic network.

Then comes the semiconscious state of the cosmic being, in which spiritual beings on earth and in the rest of creation become aware of the oneness of creation. Today, for instance, people everywhere are beginning to understand concepts like Gaia, the oneness of the organism of earth. This happens by pitta, the force of intellect, or Vishnu the preserver, who keeps a balance on earth between the spiritual and the demonic. The spiritual are those who understand the illusion, and the demonic are those who are attached to the illusion and suffer from its deception.

This illusion is explained by the old Indian story of the serpent and the rope. When the rope is mistaken for the serpent, we are frightened. However, the moment we recognize that it is a rope, that fear is removed. Similarly, the illusion of the universe creates fear arising from duality, leading to the downfall of the ego driven by demonic desire.

A PARABLE FOR
THE AYURVEDIC THEORY
OF CREATION

It is difficult to provide an illustration of such an event because it involves a compression of both human time and space.

An example of the compression of human time is provided in a story of Lord Shiva and a devotee of his, who had long prayed for Shiva's appearance before him. When, after many years, Shiva appears before him, he asks the lord what he can offer him. Shiva smiles and says he wants nothing at all from his devotee. But the devotee insists that he must offer the lord something and so Shiva says he will have a glass of water, since he insists.

The devotee goes to get water from the well in the nearby village. At the well he sees a beautiful woman whom he falls in love with, courts, and marries. He forgets all about Shiva and begins to live a family life.

After many, many years there is a big flood in the region, and as his house and all his belongings float away in the water, he suddenly remembers Shiva and the glass of water he had promised him.

When the flood waters recede, he goes with a glass of water to the spot where he had seen Shiva. Shiva is there, in deep meditation. He wakes up, takes the glass of water offered, and smiles and thanks him for bringing back the water in a "second."

This story illustrates the relationship between divine time and human time. What is a mere second for Shiva is a lifetime for man.

Likewise, the human space of earth and the solar system is compressed into a mere pimple in divine consciousness. As the cosmic consciousness moves from cosmic sleep into awareness, prakrti returns to purusha, and the illusion of this manifested universe realizes its oneness with God.

R.E.M.

God's sleep is the dream
of our existence. Neurons
of his dream crackle
an explosion of galaxies.

The birth of life is imminent, in
his next rapid eye movement.

In his dark body, as he sleeps
I see a white lotus creeping up
from the right atrium
into the throat.

He should soon awake, glowing
in pure consciousness.

The world dream will cease.

from "Karma is a Slow Virus."

GOPI WARRIER *(1982)*

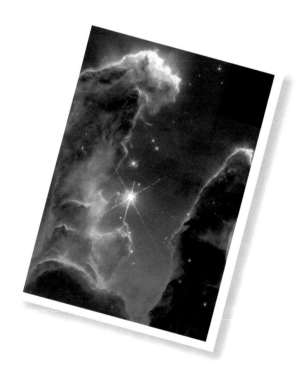

ABOVE *Pillars of gas (vata),*
trillions of miles long, both
destroying and creating new stars.

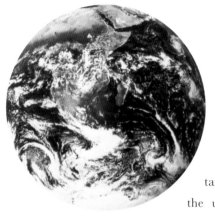

The pitta nature of Vishnu the preserver thus creates the balance of the energies between rest and activity, maintaining the illusion of the universe, but at the same time allowing the spiritually inclined within it to escape its duality. This is the universal being aware of its own dream, or reaching the end of the dream.

Eventually, the universe "ages" as cosmic vata comes into play and the destruction of dream and illusion begins. Prakrti returns into oneness with purusha, the cosmic being. At present the universe is moving into this final state.

The culmination of this process is retraction of the universe into the bindu state of consciousness – or the "black hole" – from which a new universe will emerge. The nature of the black hole is ether, or pure akasha, which retains all memories of its previous existence but is devoid of their form. In other words, it is pure consciousness without form, and the cosmic being has retracted and trapped all creation, all illusion within the light of its own evanescence.

This area is truly "Vedic space," unlike cyberspace, which is dead. Vedic space is eternal and accessible only to those initiated in the correct manner by the correct teacher because the mantras and the ritual of that initiation are the access codes to this universal being. The Vedic sages still inhabit this space, articulating the direction of the universe by the power of their mantras.

CYBERSPACE

The author proposes that cyberspace is dead space, and laden with corpses, two of which were said to have been fed into the Internet. In contrast, Vedic space is eternal and universal.

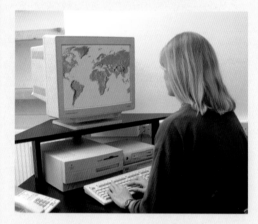

ABOVE *The cyberspace of the Internet provides "dead" knowledge, unlike revealed Vedic truth.*

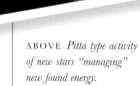

ABOVE *Pitta type activity of new stars "managing" new found energy.*

TOP LEFT *The Earth. Gaia, the Earth goddess is worshipped as Bhudevi in India.*

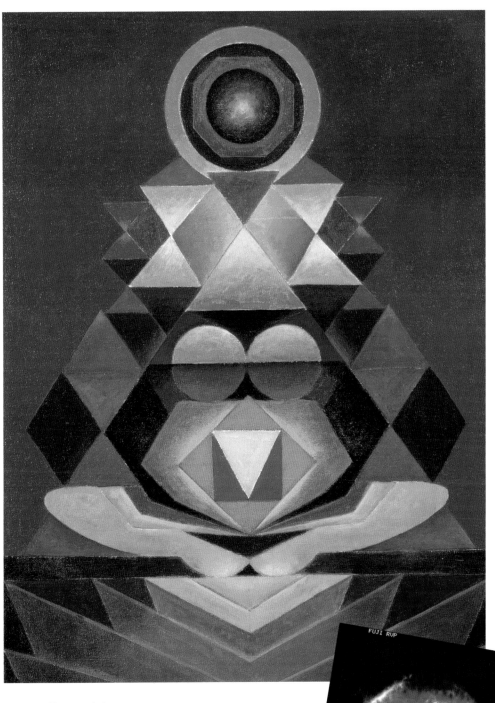

ABOVE *Abstract painting*
of cosmic being in meditation
by G. Santosh.

RIGHT *Red kapha star in*
the creative process. Red is a
sexual, procreative color.

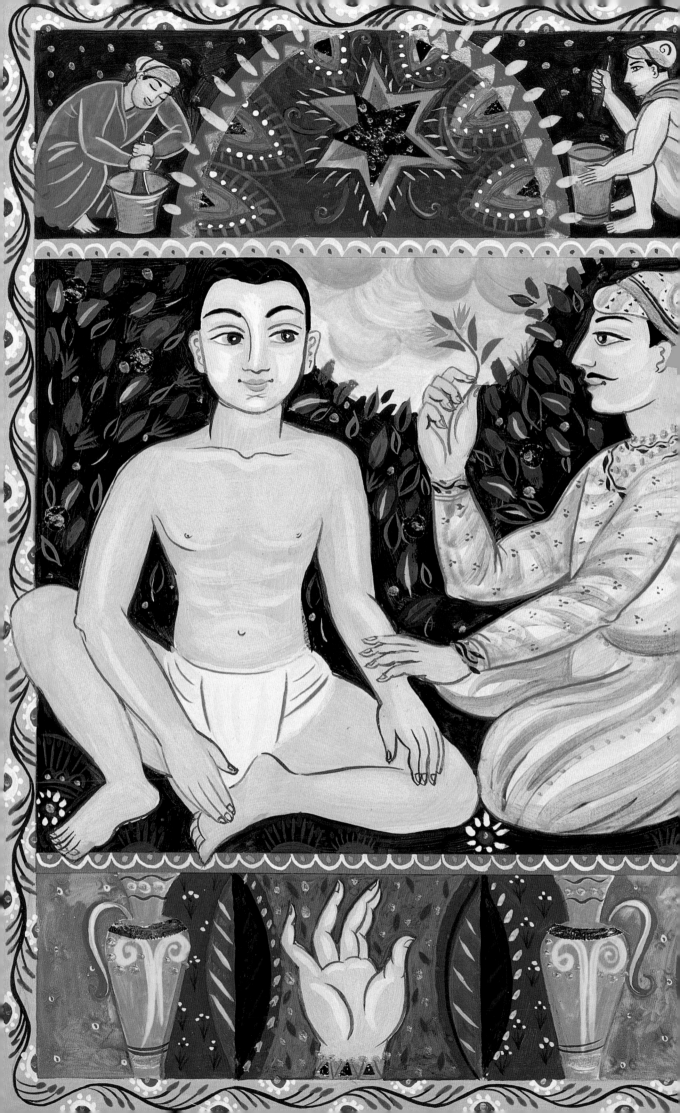

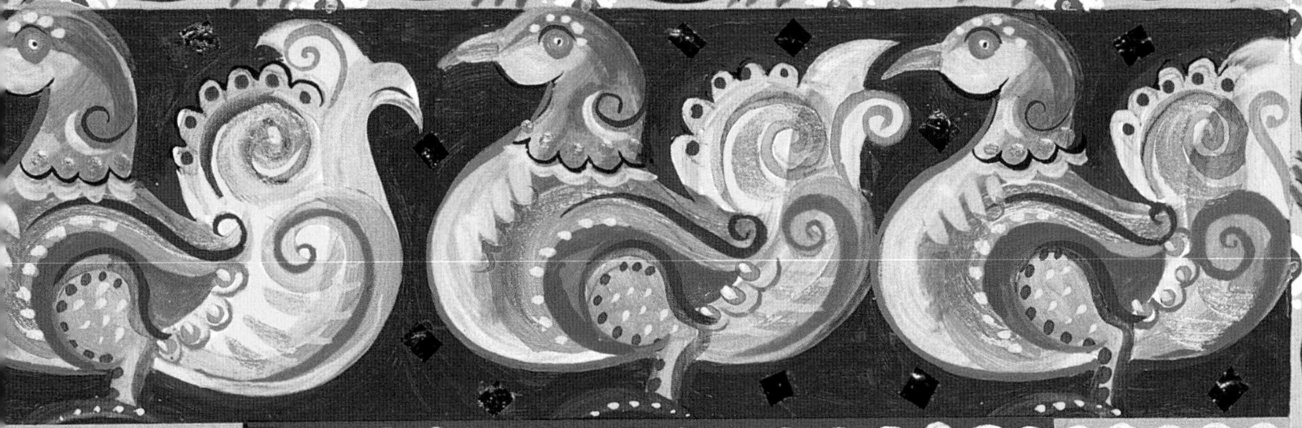

CHAPTER THREE

⟊

The Principles
of Ayurveda

IN AYURVEDIC *philosophy, everything in the
universe is composed of five elements, the
panchamahabhutas. These combine into three doshas
(the tridoshas) or bioenergetic forces that govern our health
and determine our prakrti, or physical constitution. The
three gunas — or psychic forces — determine our mental and
spiritual health. Ayurveda is a holistic system of healthcare
that teaches us to balance these energies in order to achieve
optimum health and well-being, and to preserve life.*

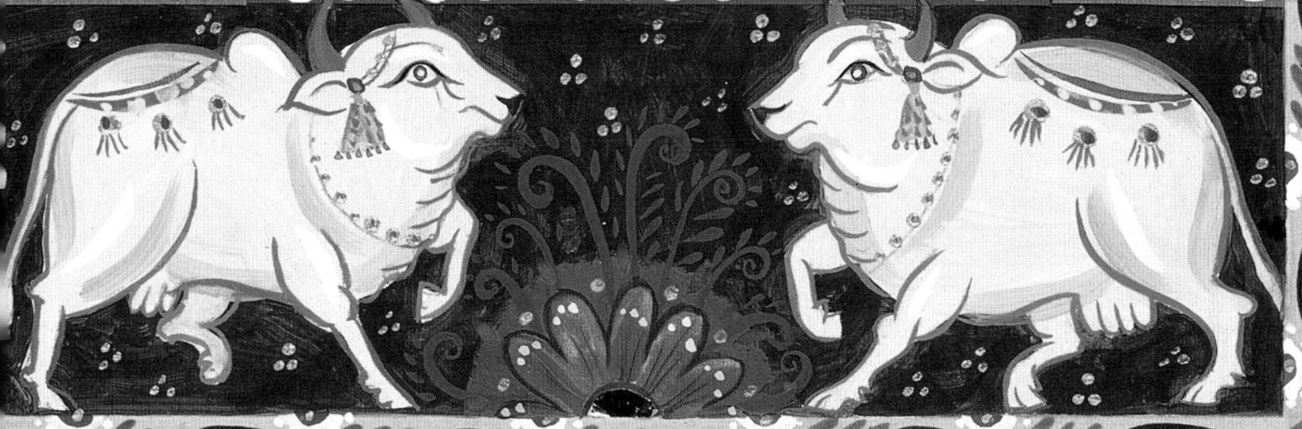

Healthy Living

T HE PRESENT definition of health by the World Health Organization (WHO) is that "Health is a state of physical, mental, and social well-being and not only the absence of disease or infirmity." This closely resembles the definition laid down in Ayurvedic texts, more than 3,000 years ago.

Sushruta, an Ayurvedic sage, defines a healthy person as "one whose doshas, agnis, dhatus, and malas (three biological units, the enzymes or digestive capacity, the tissue elements and the excretory functions) are in harmonious condition and whose mind and senses are cheerful." Today, this approach to healthy living is experiencing a renaissance as an understanding of the mind, body, and spirit relationship grows.

MAIN PILLARS

The author of ancient Ayurvedic texts Charaka wrote, "The healthy life has three main pillars – a balanced diet, proper sleep and a healthy sex life, and mental hygiene."

With the growing strains of day-to-day living and a revolution in eating habits and lifestyle, one is exposed to extremes of stress, leading to intense demands on mind and body. Stress can result from hectic daily living, inadequate nutrition, environmental pollution, and a number of other factors. This creates an imbalance in our bodies and our minds, and because they are so inextricably linked, our physical and mental ailments need to be considered simultaneously.

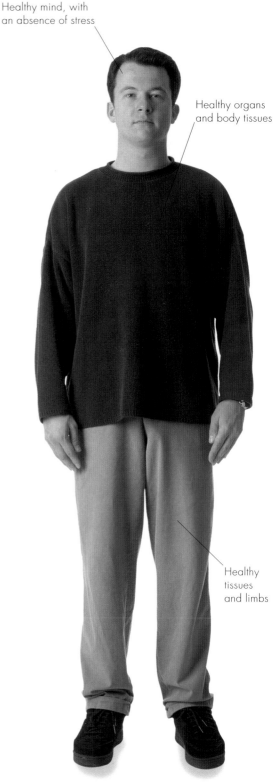

Healthy mind, with an absence of stress

Healthy organs and body tissues

Healthy tissues and limbs

ABOVE *Health is a state of physical, mental, and social well-being, and not only the absence of disease or infirmity (World Health Organization).*

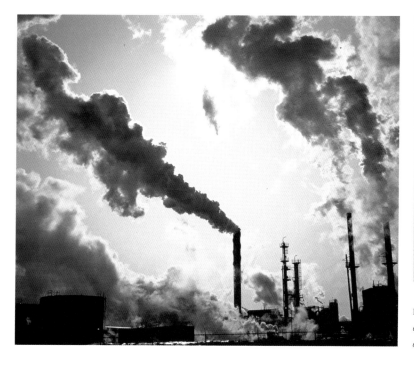

LEFT *Pollution is a major cause of disease as the natural balance of doshas in the environment is upset.*

Ayurveda takes a holistic approach. The body and the mind are both considered to be receptive to disease or well-being. Well-being is the harmonious interaction of body and mind, and disease is caused by a deficient interaction between them. The objective of Ayurveda is not only to establish the equilibrium of the three basic elements, but also to maintain this equilibrium for a disease-free state.

Illness of the body is taken care of with medication and specialized therapeutic procedures, and illness of the mind is remedied by spiritual knowledge, philosophy, concentration, and by following the rules of ethical conduct. Ayurvedic remedies and a unique medical approach are also used to treat and balance illnesses of the mind.

The emphasis on maintaining good health, or swasthavrtta, is crucial to Ayurveda. The daily routine or dinacharya, and the seasonal regimen or ritucharya are designed to keep us healthy. In dinacharya, diet, physical exercise, personal hygiene, and mental health are all important. Because it is a science of life, Ayurveda addresses every aspect of our lives, and by incorporating the daily prescriptions for good health (of the mind, body, and spirit) into our routines, we will experience optimum health and well-being (*see* Chapter Five: An Ayurvedic Lifestyle).

HOLISTIC APPROACH

Ayurveda is not a series of medicines or treatment that address symptoms or particular ailments; it is aimed at treating the whole person – the mind, body, and spirit – in order to create a balance that will ensure optimum health and also well-being.

LEFT *Yoga and meditation are important elements of a healthy lifestyle and will give a sense of physical and mental well-being.*

The Meaning of Life

LIFE IS DEFINED as the union of the body, senses, mind, and soul. According to Indian philosophy there can be no life if this combination or union does not exist. The evolution of matter in the universe takes place in a cyclic manner and involves these 24 principal elements:

- Prakrti
- Maha (intellect)
- Ahamkara (egoism)
- Manas (mind)
- Five sensory organs
- Five motor organs
- Five tanmatras (rudimentary elements)
- Five mahabhutas (physical elements)

Life is an evolutionary process that begins with the union of prakrti (the physical part of the universe) with the purusha (the spiritual part). From these, the remaining 23 elements develop to give life to the body. Throughout our lives, there is a continuous dissolution taking place. When the union of prakrti and purusha dissolves, and the 23 other elements no longer exist, the life process ends.

In Indian philosophy, the purpose of life is to achieve dharma (virtue), artha (wealth), kama (enjoyment), and moksha (salvation). To achieve this, you need a healthy state of body and mind. It is equally possible for a state of disease to exist in the body and mind as it is for well-being to exist. As discussed earlier, well-being is achieved through the balance of the biological units (tridoshas), and disease is an imbalance of these units.

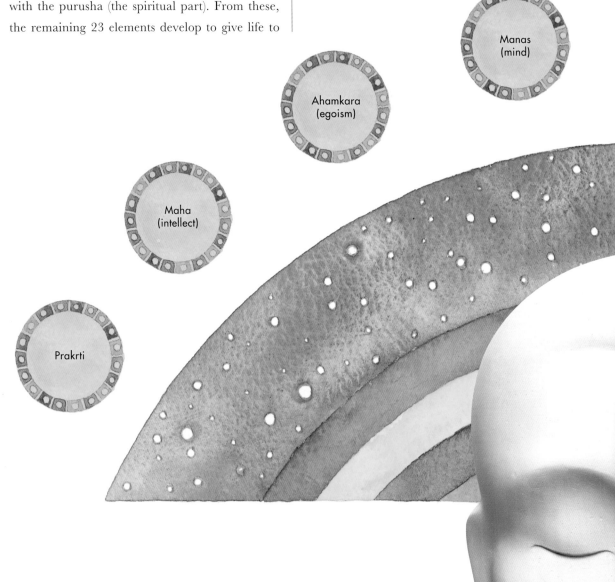

Manas
(mind)

Ahamkara
(egoism)

Maha
(intellect)

Prakrti

RESTORING THE BALANCE

The objective of Ayurveda is to reestablish equilibrium when ill and to maintain equilibrium to keep healthy.

As a science of life, Ayurveda attempts to set out good and bad practices, by outlining the causes of happy and unhappy life, and what is wholesome and unwholesome. It provides guidelines for living that are clear and provides balance to often hectic and unhealthy lifestyles.

According to Charaka, life is of four types:

- Hita (useful or creative)
- Ahita (harmful or destructive)
- Sukha (happy)
- Duhkha (unhappy or miserable)

Your life is happy when you are not afflicted with either physical or mental illness and are endowed with youth, strength, virility, knowledge, and excellent sense organs (eyes, nose, mouth, ears, and skin). You are happy when your efforts are prosperous and you are able to plan your life as you like. A life contrary to this is unhappy.

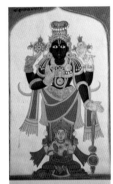

RIGHT *Lord Vishnu, the preserver of the balance between creation and destruction.*

LEFT *Well-being is achieved through the balance of the doshas.*

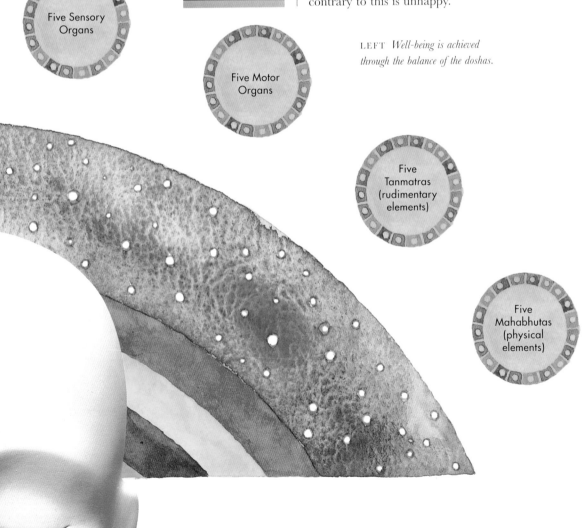

Five Sensory Organs

Five Motor Organs

Five Tanmatras (rudimentary elements)

Five Mahabhutas (physical elements)

Theory of Panchamahabhutas and the Five Elements

ACCORDING TO Ayurvedic philosophy all matter in our universe is made up of five basic eternal substances in various proportions. They are:

* Akasha (space)
* Vayu (air)
* Agni (fire)
* Jala (water)
* Prthvi (earth)

These five substances comprise the panchamahabhutas, or the five elements or eternal substances, and combine with the soul to create a living being.

All five elements exist in all things, including our bodies, and have specific qualities. Space corresponds to the spaces in the body: the mouth, nostrils, thorax, abdomen, respiratory tract, and cells. Air is the element of movement so it represents muscular movement, pulsation, the expansion and contraction of the lungs, and intestines, even the movement within every cell. Fire controls enzyme functioning. It shows itself as intelligence, fuels the digestive system, and regulates the metabolism. Water is in plasma, blood, saliva, digestive juices, the mucous membranes and cytoplasm, and the liquid inside cells. Earth manifests in the solid structures of the body: the bones, nails, teeth, muscles, cartilage, tendons, skin, and hair.

The panchamahabhutas, or five eternal substances, become intermixed in a special way in order to create various types of substances that exist in the world. Our bodies – like all other material things – are made up of these five mahabhutas, or substances, each of which has its own unique properties and actions.

PANCHABHAUTIKA PREDOMINANCE IN VARIOUS CONSTITUENTS AND ORGANS

MAHABHAUTIKA PREDOMINANCE	RELATIVE ORGANS AND FACULTIES
Akasha *Dominance of akasha mahabhuta*	Products of the nature of void such as speech and sounds emanating from different organs of the body.
Vayavya *Dominance of vayu mahabhuta*	Bodily functions like inhalation, exhalation, opening and closing of eyelids, extension and contraction of joints, locomotion and other motor functions. Factors of the body known by touch. Tactile faculty.
Agneya *Dominance of agni mahabhuta*	Factors like pitta, temperature, heat, and luster of the body colors. Visual faculty.
Apya *Dominance of jala mahabhuta*	Factors that are liquid, moving, slow, soft, smooth, oily, slimy, plasma, muscle, fat, kapha, pitta, urine, and sweat. Taste of the body. Gustatory faculty.
Parthiva *Dominance of prthvi mahabhuta*	Organs that are solid, gross, stable, having a shape and form, rough and hard such as teeth, bones, nails, flesh, skin, tendons, muscles. Body odors. Olfactory faculty.

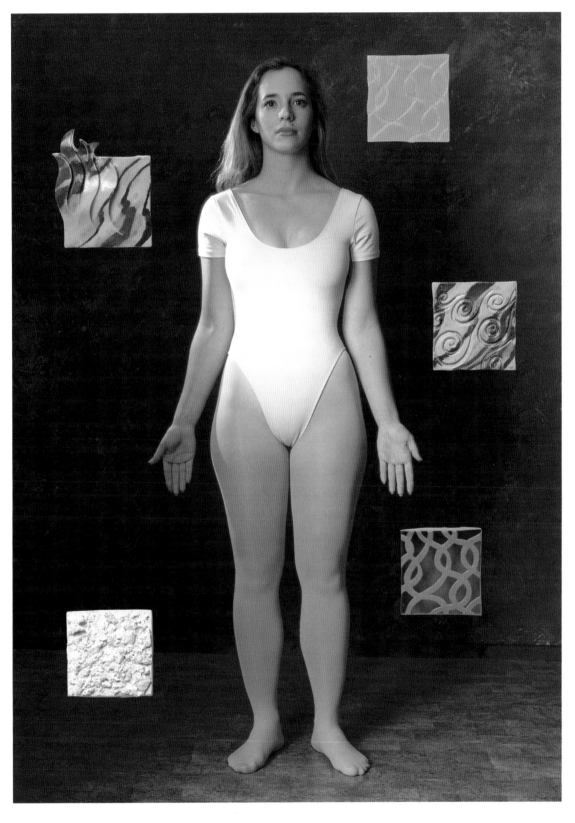

ABOVE *The five elements of the universe are replicated in our body.*

As you can see, the panchamahabhutas or five basic elements possess very specific qualities. To take it one step further, space, air, fire, water, and earth also have the following as their inherent qualities:

❀ Sabda (sound)

❀ Sparsa (touch)

❀ Rupa (sight)

❀ Rasa (taste)

❀ Gandha (smell)

Each of these qualities has to be perceived, and we have five sense organs that are uniquely developed to perform that very function for us. The relationship between the elements and the senses and sense organs is as follows – space is sound, air is touch, fire is sight, water is taste, and, lastly, earth is smell. The vocal chords, hands, feet, genitals, and anus are also related to these organs. So too are their functions of talking, holding, moving, procreating, and excreting.

The combination of elements creates the three doshas (tridoshas) in the following way: vata governs air and space; pitta governs fire and water; kapha governs water and earth.

Karma from previous lives dictates the doshic pakrti of the individual and this in turn governs the genetic make-up. The vasanas (desires) latent in an individual due to karma make them pursue lifestyles that exacerbate the doshas and this can then result in disease.

GLOSSARY

Bhuta

The five eternal substances, or panchamahabhutas, are individually referred to as bhuta. The five bhutas – space, air, fire, water, and earth – combine to form the panchamahabhutas.

Panchamahabhutas

The five basic eternal substances – akasha (space), vayu (air), agni (fire), jala (water), and prthvi (earth). The Ayurveda theory of creation believes these five eternal substances to be responsible for the creation of all living beings.

PROPERTIES AND ACTIONS OF THE FIVE ELEMENTS

PANCHAMAHABHUTAS	PROPERTIES	ACTIONS
Space *Akasha*	Smooth, soft, subtle, porous, non-slimy, property of sound, and no distinct taste.	Produces softness, lightness, and porosity.
Air *Vayu*	Rough, light, dry, cold, soluble. Property of touch, largely astringent and slightly bitter in taste.	Removes sliminess, produces lightness, dryness, and emaciation.
Fire *Agni*	Heat-producing, pungent, rough, bright, attribute of form, pungent taste.	Produces burning sensation, helps digestion and maturation. Increases temperature. Improves eyesight.
Water *Jala*	Cold, fluid, heavy, moist, slowly digested, slimy, having property of taste, sweet with astringent, sour, and saline taste.	Imparts glossiness, produces moisture. Increases fluid content. Acts as nutritive, emollient, and purgative.
Earth *Prthvi*	Heavy, firm, immobile, dull, compact, thick, strong, rough, having sweet taste.	Increases firmness, strength, hardness of body, emollient, nutritive, and purgative.

THE FIVE ELEMENTS AND THE FIVE SENSES

PANCHAMAHABHUTAS	QUALITIES	SENSE ORGANS	SENSORY FACULTIES
	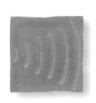		
Space *Akasha*	Sound *Sabda*	Ears	Auditory
Air *Vayu*	Touch *Sparsa*	Skin	Tactual

Fire *Agni*	Sight *Rupa*	Eyes	Visual

Water *Jala*	Taste *Rasa*	Tongue	Gustatory
Earth *Prthvi*	Smell *Gandha*	Nose	Olfactory

The Tridoshas

THE TRIDOSHAS (or three doshas) are the primary and essential factors of the human body that govern our entire physical structure and function. They are called vata, pitta, and kapha, and they are derived from the five basic eternal substances, the panchamahabhutas. Each dosha has a predominance of one of the five bhutas.

Vata consists of the combined predominance of vayu and akasha (air and space). Pitta consists of tejas and jala (fire and water), and kapha is formed by jala and prthvi (water and earth).

When we are healthy, our three doshas are in balance, or in a state of equilibrium. The tridoshas in their normal, balanced state give us strength, a good complexion, normal functioning of the vital organs, and long life. When the three doshas are imbalanced, disease is caused.

Each of the doshas has its subtypes, possessing properties that perform various functions at different levels of our individual bodies.

Many of the physical and mental phenomena ascribed to the nervous system by modern physiology can be identified with vata. Similarly, the entire chemical process operating in your body can be attributed to pitta, including enzymes, hormones, and the complete nutritional system. The activities of the skeletal and anabolic system (those aspects of the metabolism involved in constructing the physical body) can be attributed to kapha – suggesting that the entire physical volume in a living organism is in fact a result of kapha.

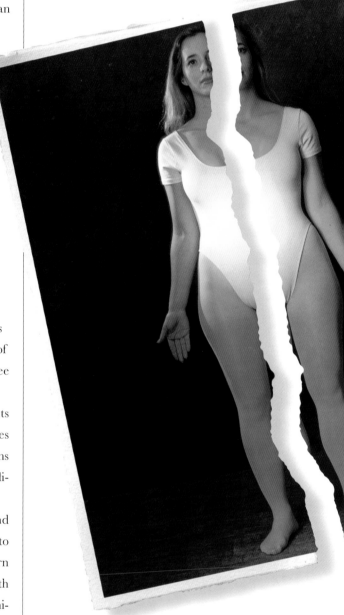

In other words, the entire constructive process in a living organism can be attributed to kapha; the entire chemical process to pitta; and the sensory and motor activities (movement) to vata.

LEFT *Lord Vishnu, in the form of "Balaji." In this form he integrates the male and female principles.*

ABOVE *When we are healthy, our three doshas are in a state of equilibrium. Unbalanced doshas cause ill health.*

THE THREE DOSHAS AND THEIR COMPOSITION

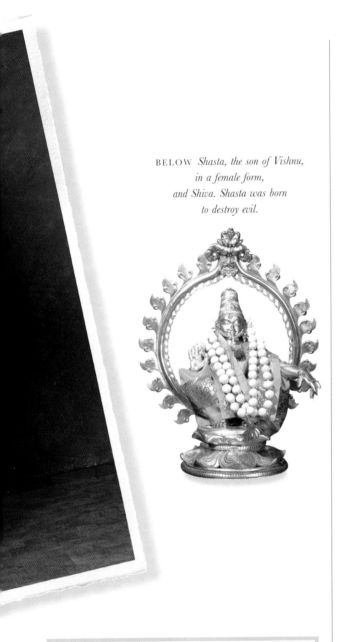

BELOW *Shasta, the son of Vishnu, in a female form, and Shiva. Shasta was born to destroy evil.*

VATA

Vayu *(air)* and akasha *(space)*

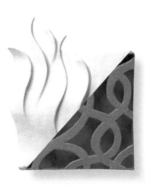

PITTA

Tejas *(fire)* and jala *(water)*

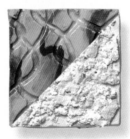

KAPHA

Jala *(water)* and prthvi *(earth)*

WHOLENESS

Charaka, the great Ayurvedic sage, explained: "Vata, pitta, and kapha maintain the integrity of the living human organism in their normal state and combine as to make the man a complete being with his indriyas (sense organs) possessed of strength, good complexion, and assured of longevity."

Vata

Vata is a Sanskrit word meaning "to move," or "to enthuse." Vata forms the most important constituent of the tridoshic framework and has a predominance of akasha and vayu (space and air) mahabhutas (*see* page 44). It is responsible for the movements of the body (both physical and mental). It upholds all the supportive structure and tissue, and governs circulation throughout the body.

The physical properties of vata have been described as:

- Ruksha (dry)
- Laghu (light)
- Site (cold)
- Suksma (subtle)
- Chala (unstable)
- Khara (rough)
- Visada (clear and transparent)

Each of these physical properties or qualities of vata stems from your intra-uterine life – that is, life in the womb – which determines your individual prakrti, or physical constitution.

Normally, vata is responsible for the entire physiological functioning of your body. It also regulates

your mind and its functioning. Thus, when vata is unbalanced, you are likely to suffer from various psychosomatic disturbances. It causes loss of weight and strength, and gives rise to emotions like anxiety, worry, grief, fear, and anger.

CHARAKA ON VATA

Charaka described the following functions of vata:

- **Enthusiasm**
- **Process of inspiration and expiration**
- **Actions or movements like walking, talking, and lifting**
- **Circulation of the supporting elements, in particular rasa (lymph) and rakta (blood)**
- **Elimination of various discharges from the body**

RIGHT *Rheumatoid arthritis is a disease caused by aggravated vata.*

FUNCTIONS OF VATA

The functions attributed to vata are extensively described by both Charaka and Sushruta.

According to Sushruta, vata is responsible for:

- **Imparting motion to the body (praspandanam)**
- **Conducting impulses from respective sense organs (udvahanam)**
- **Separating egesta, which is waste, from ingested food (virek)**
- **Retaining and evacuating urine and semen (dharanam)**

AIR

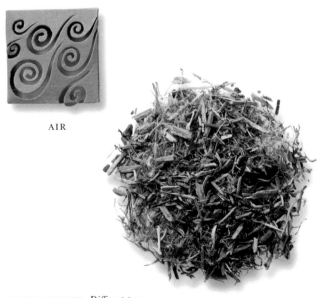

ABOVE RIGHT *Different teas are recommended for different individuals. This is a vata type.*

Sites and types of vata

Vata exists in these five forms according to its function and the site of activity:

- Prana
- Udana
- Vyana
- Samana
- Apana

Disturbed vata

When the balance of vata is disturbed, it brings about:

- Rheumatic and joint pain
- Arthritis
- Constipation
- Abnormal blood pressure and heart disease
- Mental instability

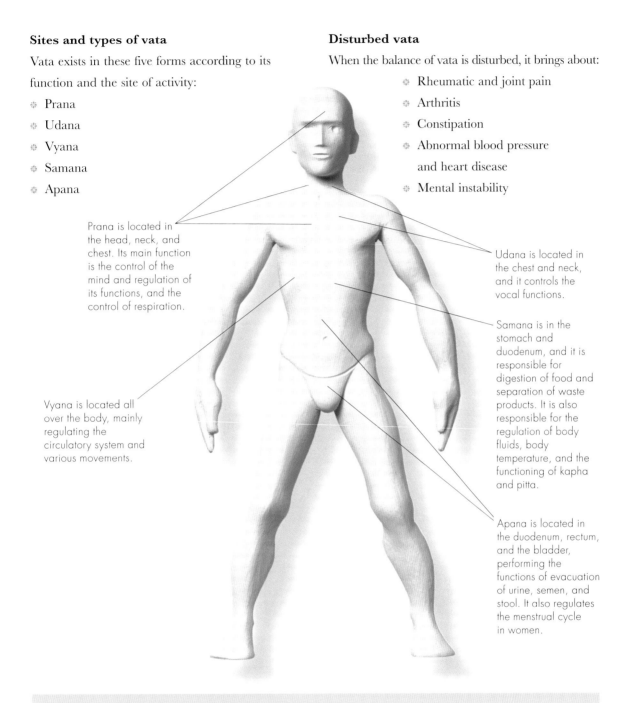

Prana is located in the head, neck, and chest. Its main function is the control of the mind and regulation of its functions, and the control of respiration.

Vyana is located all over the body, mainly regulating the circulatory system and various movements.

Udana is located in the chest and neck, and it controls the vocal functions.

Samana is in the stomach and duodenum, and it is responsible for digestion of food and separation of waste products. It is also responsible for the regulation of body fluids, body temperature, and the functioning of kapha and pitta.

Apana is located in the duodenum, rectum, and the bladder, performing the functions of evacuation of urine, semen, and stool. It also regulates the menstrual cycle in women.

VATA CHARACTERISTICS

❖ Vata, which is rough, cool, light, subtle, mobile, non-slimy and coarse, is balanced by medicines with opposite qualities.

❖ Vata people have restless minds and weak memories. They avoid confrontation. They have active and sensitive natures and express themselves through sport and creative pursuits, and sometimes by overindulgence in pleasures. They are the most eager for sexual activity among the three prakrtis.

❖ Vata is the strongest of the doshas and its powerful, mobile nature is spread across the sensory organs, the entire nervous system, and the tissues, carrying nourishment, separating nutrients from waste products, and operating the respiratory system.

Pitta

Pitta is a Sanskrit word meaning "to heat" or "to burn." Pitta is responsible for all biochemical activities, including the production of heat. Pitta is comprised of fire (tejas) and water (jala).

The inherent natural qualities of pitta are:

- Heat (ushma)
- Sharpness (teekshna)
- Liquidity (drav)
- Slight oiliness (sneham)
- Blue and yellow colors (neelpitta)
- Fleshy and unpleasant smell (pichhila)
- Acrid and sour tastes (amlam)
- Fluidity (sara)

Your individual constitution or prakrti has features that are similar to these natural qualities. In diseases too, the natural qualities and actions of pitta are often wholly or partially present.

RIGHT *This is a pitta type of tea. Pitta individuals should drink this variety.*

> ## FUNCTIONS OF PITTA
>
> **The functions of pitta include:**
> - **Vision**
> - **Digestion**
> - **Heat production**
> - **Imparting of color to the body**
> - **Hunger, thirst, and appetite**
> - **Softness and suppleness of the body**
> - **All intellectual functions**

> ## ROYAL PITTA
>
> *There is an ancient saying in Ayurveda that the kapha person should be treated like an enemy, the vata person like a friend and an enemy, and the pitta person like a king!*

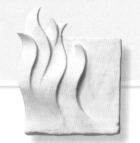

FIRE

TYPES OF PITTA

FORMS OF PITTA	EFFECTS IN THE NORMAL STATE	EFFECTS IN AN ABNORMAL STATE
Pacaka pitta	Digestion	Indigestion
Alochaka pitta	Vision	Impaired vision, or loss of vision
Bhrajaka pitta	Normal body heat, normal complexion	Abnormal body heat, abnormal complexion
Sadhaka pitta	Happiness, joy, and valor	Fear, anger, and bewilderment
Ranjaka pitta	Healthy blood formation	Deficient blood formation

Sites and types of pitta

Pitta has been classified into five types:

- Alochaka
- Sadhaka
- Bhrajaka
- Pacaka
- Ranjaka

Alochaka pitta is located in the eyes and is responsible for normal vision and the color of the eyes.

Bhrajaka pitta is present in the skin of the entire body, and it imparts color and luster to the skin while maintaining the normal body temperature.

Ranjaka pitta is located in the liver and spleen and is responsible for the formation of blood and for giving color to lymphatic fluid, which runs through our lymphatic system and forms the basis of immunity.

Disturbed pitta

When the balance of pitta is disturbed, it brings about:

- Impaired visual perception
- Burning sensations all over the body
- Abnormal or subnormal temperature
  - Impaired skin health, luster, color, and complexion
  - Confused mind and anger
  - Yellowness of urine, feces, eyes, and skin

Sadhaka pitta is located in the heart and is responsible for intelligence, memory, and enthusiasm. According to Sushruta, the heart is the seat of consciousness, which is responsible for the functions of the brain.

Pacaka pitta is located in the stomach and duodenum and is responsible for proper digestion and assimilation.

PITTA CHARACTERISTICS

❖ Pitta, which is hot, sharp, liquid, sour, fluid, and pungent, is balanced by medicines that have the opposite qualities.

❖ Pittas have an intellectual, precise, and irritable disposition. They are articulate, learned, and proud. They tend to gray soon. They have hot, sweaty bodies.

❖ Their eyes get red in the summer and after bathing, and they are sharp and knifelike in anger. They have an aggressive nature.

❖ Pitta provides color, shine, and heat to the body and creates intellect, awareness, vision, hunger, thirst, and taste to the human constitution.

Kapha

Kapha is a Sanskrit word meaning "phlegm," but also "to embrace" or "to keep together." Kapha is a source of strength and resistance (bolla). According to Ayurveda, kapha is responsible for the construction of the living body, and it is made up of the water and earth elements (jala and prthvi). Due to its composition, kapha is more stable in nature than the other two doshas. Kapha in its normal state is responsible for the strength and formation of the body.

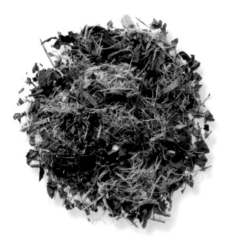

ABOVE *It is recommended that kapha people drink teas specially prepared for their type.*

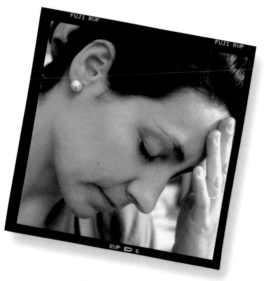

ABOVE *Aggravated kapha with obstructed vata causes sinus headaches and migraines.*

Physical characteristics of Kapha are described as:

* Guru (heavy)
* Sita (cool)
* Mirdu (soft)
* Ishat (viscous)
* Madhura (sweet)
* Sthira (stable)
* Picchila (slimy)

Kapha brings about:

* Sturdiness
* Plumpness
* Enthusiasm
* Wisdom
* Virility

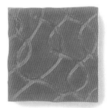

WATER

FUNCTIONS OF KAPHA

The main functions of kapha are:

* Maintaining oiliness of the body and organs
* Maintaining general stability of the body
* Providing excellent strength, patience, and virility
* Promoting smooth working of joints
* Forbearance
* Courage
* Generosity

Your body's bulk, compactness, and physical strength are also due to kapha.

Sites and types of kapha

Kapha is of five types, depending upon their site and function:

- Tarpaka
- Bodhaka
- Avalambaka
- Kledaka
- Sleshmaka

Tarpaka kapha is in the head, and helps the brain and the sensory organs to perform their specific functions in the body.

Bodhaka kapha is in the tongue and pharynx, and it enables us to perceive taste.

Kledaka kapha is located in the stomach (amashaya). It moistens the food, and after breakdown of food particles into smaller ones, it liquefies the stomach contents.

Disturbed kapha

When the balance of kapha is disturbed, it brings about:

- Emaciation of the body
- Loss of oiliness
- Flabbiness
- Weakness and susceptibility to disease
- Impotence and sterility
- Immobility and loss of function of the joints
- Weariness and lethargy
- Confusion, ignorance, and lack of understanding

Avalambaka kapha is located in the heart and sternal region (hrdaya and trika). Its function is to support and nourish the heart.

Sleshmaka kapha is in all the bony joints of the body and its main function is to protect the joints and keep them lubricated, firm, and united, thus maintaining their smooth functioning.

KAPHA CHARACTERISTICS

- ❖ Kapha, which is heavy, cool, soft, oily, sweet, immobile, and slimy, is relieved by medicines with the opposite qualities.
- ❖ Kapha people have stable, patient personalities and are slow to anger. They are not easily provoked but, once angry, do not easily calm down.

- ❖ They are honorable, keep their word, and avoid lies.
- ❖ They are inclined to be slow talkers, and can be lethargic, even lazy, if not driven by others.
- ❖ Kapha gives strength, softness, contentment, peace, and satisfaction, and is the primary agent of all cellular development and reproductive activity within the body.

Behavior and the Tridoshas

A number of the common ailments and chronic conditions affecting us in middle and old age are the result of behavioral and emotional patterns that have evolved in our modern world. We are creatures of habit, and much of our behavior is based on beliefs that have been passed through generations without any sensible basis.

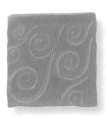

AIR

For example, in the Western world there is a commonly held belief that fresh air is good for us. On one level this is true, balance must be maintained in our lives and that means experiencing all five elements. It does not mean that you have to be exposed to extremely cold winter air without sufficient protection for long periods of time.

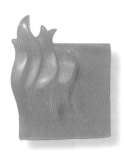

FIRE

Such exposure to cold can eventually give rise to arthritis and rheumatism, conditions that manifest themselves later in life. Many young people do not seem to feel the cold, and go out in short sleeves or with only a suit in winter or late fall. For a vata prakrti individual (a person with a vata constitution, *see* page 48) this persistent behavior will undoubtedly lead to aggravation of vata, which will cause conditions like arthritis and rheumatism.

Behavior that aggravates vata includes:
- Too many late nights, causing excessive fatigue and nervous strain
- Too much dancing or aerobic activity
- Too much running and other exercise due to an obsessive desire to lose weight

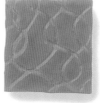

WATER

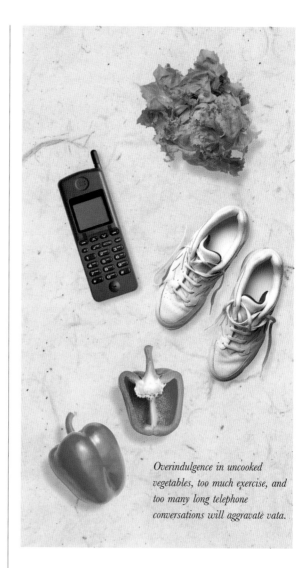

Overindulgence in uncooked vegetables, too much exercise, and too many long telephone conversations will aggravate vata.

- Overindulgence in leafy vegetables, or uncooked vegetables or food
- Excessive sexual indulgence
- Too many long telephone conversations, particularly on mobile telephones
- Insufficient time alone or in meditation
- Watching too many videos or movies, or too much television
- Too many emotionally charged relationships without sufficient time to feel, and think through them
- Lack of emotional or family support
- Lack of touch
- Absence of routine

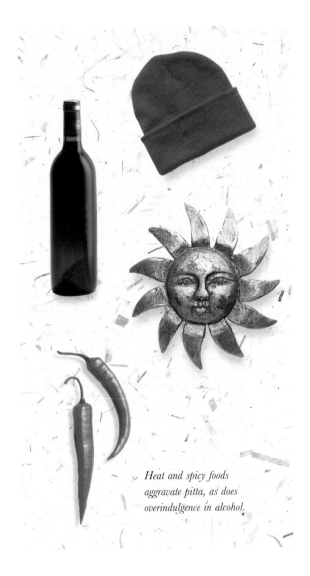

Heat and spicy foods aggravate pitta, as does overindulgence in alcohol.

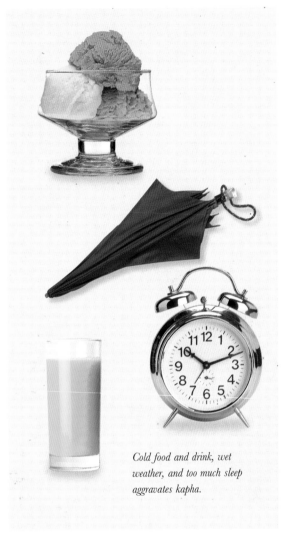

Cold food and drink, wet weather, and too much sleep aggravates kapha.

Behavior that aggravates pitta includes:

- Too much exposure to the sun in summer
- Wearing too many clothes in the summer, e.g., thick suits and ties
- Indulgence in too much spicy food
- Excessive intake of alcohol
- Insufficient intake of water, particularly in summer
- Indulgence in too many arguments
- Too few outdoor activities, particularly in green fields and by rivers
- Lack of a firm, loving, and secure relationship where there is no room for jealousy or competition

Behavior that aggravates kapha includes:

- Insufficient exercise
- Indolent lifestyle
- Overindulgence in sweet foods and drinks
- Too much sleep, particularly in late morning and afternoon
- Overeating, particularly rich food
- Overindulgence in cold foods, particularly ice cream, and cold drinks
- Getting wet in the rain or snow
- Wearing damp clothes, or not drying properly after a shower or bath
- Excessive dependence on a loving relationship without sufficient detachment

Diseases Caused by Abnormal Doshas

The three doshas – vata, pitta, and kapha – are responsible for health and disease. When they are in balance and in a normal state they bring about good health, growth, strength, complexion, mental stability, and happiness. When the three doshas are unbalanced, or in an abnormal state, they cause various types of disease. Unbalanced vata is the most powerful, and causes many major ailments.

Unbalanced vata causes rheumatism, arthritis, musculoskeletal pain, circulatory problems, stomach pain, and constipation.

Unbalanced pitta causes acidity, skin eruptions, irritability, anger, and hysteria.

Unbalanced kapha causes obesity, drowsiness, nausea, bronchitis, asthma, heaviness in the head, and loss of memory.

TYPES OF DISEASE

There are 80 types of disease caused by abnormal vata; 40 types of disease caused by abnormal pitta; and 20 types of disease caused by abnormal kapha.

Diseases caused by unbalanced vata:

- Nakhabheda (cracking of the nails)
- Vipadika (cracking of the feet)
- Padasula (pain in the feet)
- Padabhramsa (fallen arches)
- Padasuptata (numbness of the feet)
- Vatakhuddata (clubfoot)
- Gulphagraha (stiffness of the ankle)
- Pindikodvestana (cramps in the calf)
- Grdhrasi (sciatica)
- Janubheda (genu varum – "knock-knees," where the feet are turned inward)
- Januvislesha (genu valgum – club feet where the feet are turned outward)
- Urustambha (stiffness of the thigh)
- Urusada (pain in the thigh)
- Pangulya (paraplegia)
- Gudabhramsa (rectal prolapse)
- Gudarti (tenesmus, a bowel disorder)
- Vrsanaksepa (scrotal pain)
- Sephastambha (priapism)
- Vanksananaha (groin tension)
- Sroni bheda (pelvic girdle pain)
- Vidbheda (diarrhea)
- Udavarta (misperistalsis – difficulty with passing food down into the gut)
- Khanjatva (lameness)
- Kubjatva (kyphosis – curvature of the spine)
- Vamanatva (dwarfism)
- Trikagraha (sacroiliac arthritis)
- Prasthagraha (stiffness of the back)
- Parsvamarda (chest pain)
- Udaravesta (gripping abdominal pain)
- Hrnmoha (bradycardia – slowness of heartbeat)
- Hrddrava (tachycardia – rapidity of heartbeat)
- Vaksa uddharsa (friction pain in the chest)
- Vaksa uparodha (impaired thoracic movements)
- Vaksastoda (stabbing pain in the chest)

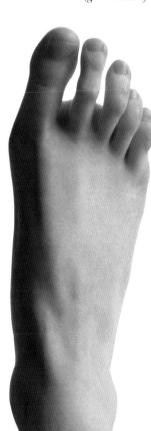

LEFT *Many foot diseases are caused by imbalanced vata, including fallen arches, stiff ankles, and cracking of the nails.*

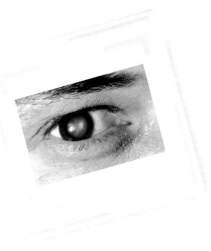

LEFT *Abnormal vata may cause eye pain.*

* Bahusosa *(atrophy of the arm)*
* Grivastambha *(stiff neck)*
* Manyastambha
  (torticollis – twisted neck)
* Kanthoddhvamsa *(hoarseness)*
* Hanubheda *(pain in the jaw)*
* Osthabheda *(pain in the hip)*
* Aksibheda *(eye pain)*
* Dantabheda *(toothache)*
* Dantasaithilya *(loose teeth)*
* Mukatva
  (aphasia – loss of speech)

* Vaksanga *(slow speech)*
* Kasayasyata
  (astringent taste in the mouth)
* Mukhasosa *(dry mouth)*
* Arasajnata
  (ageustia – loss of the sense of taste)
* Ghrananasa *(anosmia – loss of
  the sense of smell)*
* Kanasula *(earache)*
* Asabdasravana *(tinnitus)*
* Uccaihsruti *(hard of hearing)*
* Badhirya *(deafness)*
* Vartmastabha
  (ptosis – drooping of the eyelids)
* Vartmasamkoca *(entropion –
  introversion of the eyelids)*
* Timira *(cataract)*
* Aksisula
  (pinching pain in the eye)
* Aksivyudasa *(sunken eyeball)*
* Bhruvyudasa
  (drooping of the eyebrow)
* Sankhabheda *(temporal pain)*
* Lalatabheda *(frontal pain)*
* Siroruk *(headache)*
* Kesabhumisphutana *(dandruff)*
* Ardita *(facial paralysis)*
* Ekangaroga *(monoplegia –
  paralysis of one limb)*

* Sarvangaroga *(polyplegia –
  paralysis of all limbs)*
* Paksavadha *(hemiplegia – half
  body paralysis)*
* Aksepaka *(violent muscular
  convulsion, as in "clonic" fits
  in epilepsy)*
* Dandaka *(continuous muscular
  convulsion, as in "tonic" fits
  in epilepsy)*
* Tama *(fainting)*
* Bhrama *(giddiness)*
* Vepathu *(tremor)*
* Jrmbha *(yawning)*
* Hikka *(hiccup)*
* Visada *(weakness)*
* Atipralapa *(delirium)*
* Rauksya and Parusya
  (dryness and hardness)
* Syavarunavadhasata
  (dusky red appearance)
* Asvapna *(sleeplessness)*
* Anavasthitacittatva
  (mental instability)

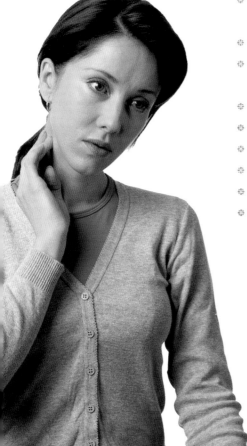

LEFT *A stiff neck is one of the many ailments that may be caused by aggravated vata.*

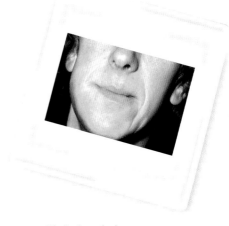

ABOVE *Toothache and other mouth problems, including abscesses, are caused by imbalanced vata.*

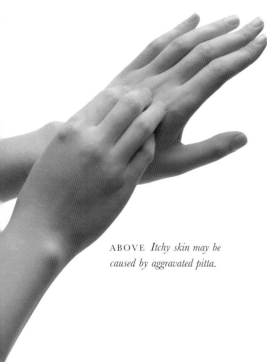

ABOVE *Itchy skin may be caused by aggravated pitta.*

Diseases caused by unbalanced pitta:

- Osa *(heat)*
- Plosa *(scorching)*
- Daha *(burning)*
- Davathu *(boiling)*
- Dhumaka *(fuming)*
- Amlaka *(acid eructation)*
- Vidaha *(burning sensation in the chest)*
- Antardaha *(burning sensation in the body)*
- Amsadaha *(burning sensation in the shoulder)*
- Usmadhikya *(high temperature)*
- Atisveda *(excessive perspiration)*
- Angagandha *(foul odor of the body)*
- Angavadarana *(cracking pain in the body)*
- Sonitakleda *(sloughing of the blood)*
- Mamsakleda *(sloughing of the muscle)*
- Tvagdaha *(burning sensation of the skin)*
- Tvagavadarana *(cracking of the skin)*

- Carmadalana *(itching of the skin)*
- Raktakoshtha *(urticaria)*
- Raktavisphota *(red vesicles)*
- Raktapitta *(bleeding tendency)*
- Rakta mandala *(red wheals)*
- Haritatva *(greenishness)*
- Kaksa *(genital herpes)*
- Kamala *(jaundice)*
- Tiktasyata *(bitter taste)*
- Lohita gandhasyata *(smell of blood from the mouth)*
- Haridratva *(icterus, jaundice)*
- Putimukhata *(foul odor of the mouth)*
- Trsnadhikya *(excessive thirst)*

- Atrpti *(dissatisfaction)*
- Asyavipaka *(stomatitis – inflammation of the lining of the mouth)*
- Galapaka *(pharyngitis)*
- Aksipaka *(conjunctivitis)*
- Gudapaka *(proctitis – inflammation of the anus)*
- Medhrapaka *(inflammation of the penis)*
- Jivadana *(hemorrhage)*
- Tamahpravesa *(fainting)*
- Haritaharidra netra, mutra, purish *(greenish yellow coloration of the eyes, urine, and feces)*
- Miluca *(skin warts)*

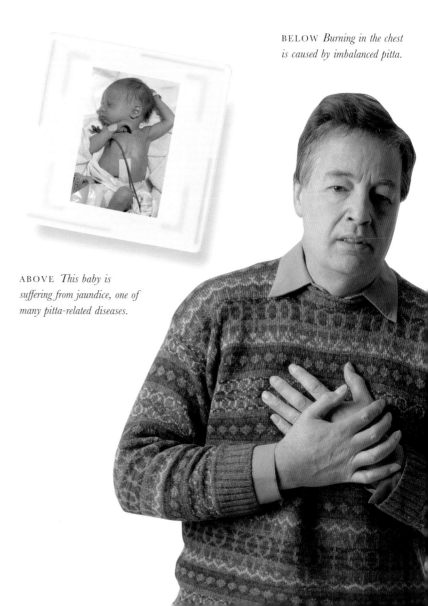

ABOVE *This baby is suffering from jaundice, one of many pitta-related diseases.*

BELOW *Burning in the chest is caused by imbalanced pitta.*

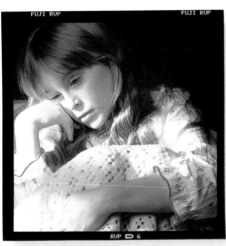

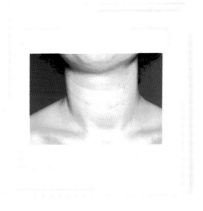

Diseases caused by unbalanced kapha:

* Trpti *(anorexia nervosa)*
* Tandra *(drowsiness)*
* Nidradhikya *(excessive sleep)*
* Staimitya *(timidity)*
* Gurugatrata
  (heaviness of the body)
* Alasya *(laziness)*
* Mukhamadhurya
  (sweet taste in the mouth)
* Mukhasrava *(salivation)*
* Slesmodgirana
  (excess mucus production)
* Maladhikya
  (excess bodily excretion)
* Balasaka *(loss of strength)*
* Apakti *(indigestion)*
* Hrdayopalepa
  (mucus around the heart)

* Kanthopalepa
  (mucus in the throat)
* Dhamanipraticaya
  (atherosclerosis – narrowing of the arteries)
* Galaganda *(goiter)*

* Atisthaulya *(obesity)*
* Sitagnita
  (suppressed digestive power)
* Udarda *(urticaria - inflammation and irritation of the skin)*
* Svetavabhasata *(pallor)*

RIGHT *Obesity is often kapha-related.*

ABOVE *This young boy is suffering from a goiter, one of the kapha-related diseases.*

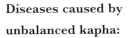

ABOVE *Laziness is both aggravated and caused by kapha.*

The Three Gunas –
Sattva, Rajas, and Tamas

JUST AS the three doshas are the essential components of your body, the three gunas – sattva, rajas, and tamas – are the three essential components of your mind. Ayurveda provides a distinct description of people on the basis of their psychological characteristics, or manasa prakrti (psychological constitution).

These psychological characteristics are genetically determined, and depend on the relative dominance of the three gunas.

All individuals have mixed amounts of these three properties, or gunas, but one predominant guna determines an individual's manasa prakrti as sattvika, rajasika, or tamasika prakrti.

When in equilibrium, sattva, rajas, and tamas – the three gunas – preserve your mind (and indirectly your body), keeping it in a healthy state. If there is a disturbance in their equilibrium, various types of mental disorders are produced.

On a mental level, rajas and tamas are comparable to the doshas in that they can be unbalanced by stress and negative desires, such as lust (kama), malice (irsya), delusion and hallucination (moha), greed (lobha), anxiety (cinta), fear (bhaya), and anger (krodha).

The general qualities have been described elsewhere. Each of the three properties is also comprised of subtypes, and the particular subtype to which a person belongs will determine the qualities of that individual.

IMBALANCE

Disturbance is caused by imbalances of rajas and tamas, since sattva is pure and is not disturbed in any way.

SATTVA

❖ Sattva is characterized by lightness, consciousness, pleasure, and clarity, and is free from disease. The senses are active because of its presence. It is also responsible for the perception of knowledge.

Psychological characteristics are genetically determined.

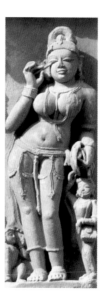

ABOVE *Stress and negative desires, such as lust, may cause imbalanced gunas.*

RAJAS

❖ Rajas is the most active of the gunas, and motion and stimulation are its characteristics. All desires, wishes, ambitions, and fickle-mindedness are a result of rajas. Various psychiatric illnesses are produced by an imbalance of rajas.

TAMAS

❖ The main characteristics of tamas are heaviness and resistance. It produces disturbances in the process of perception and activities of the mind. Delusion, false knowledge, laziness, apathy, sleep, and drowsiness are due to tamas.

LEFT *Your psychological character is determined by the relative dominance of one of the three gunas.*

RIGHT *Sattvika individuals are pure in love and thoughts. They do not perform mean acts, or suffer from jealousy or other negative desires.*

A predominant guna determines a person's psychological prakrti.

When in equilibrium, the three gunas keep mind and body healthy.

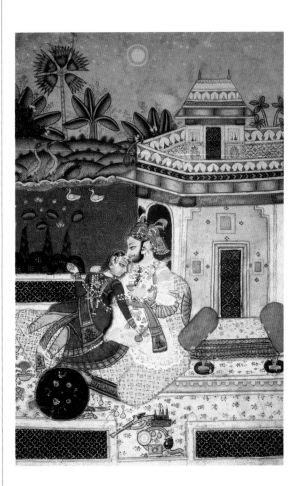

BALANCE

The role of sattva is always to maintain balance or equilibrium.

Sattvika Individuals

The sattvika person has seven subtypes:

- Brahma sattva
- Arsa sattva
- Aindra sattva
- Yamya sattva
- Varuna sattva
- Kabera sattva
- Gandharva sattva

Of these seven subtypes, brahma sattva is considered the best because it possesses knowledge, the most important quality. The other types will seem obnoxious to modern man. The vedic seers set very high standards and foresaw the inevitable downward mutation of the species in Kali yuga.

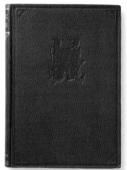

LEFT *Sattvika individuals love all knowledge, but spiritual knowledge in particular.*

BELOW *Sattvika people are truly generous and like to give.*

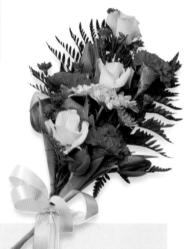

SATTVIKA SUBTYPES

SUBTYPES	QUALITIES
Brahma sattva	Free from passion, anger, greed, ignorance, or jealousy. Possessing knowledge and the power of discrimination.
Arsa sattva	Excellent memory, purity, love, and self-control. Excellent intellectual frame of mind. Free from pride, ego, ignorance, greed, or anger. Possessing the power of understanding and retention.
Aindra sattva	Devotion to sacred books, study rituals, and oblations. Devotion to virtuous acts, farsightedness, and courage. Authoritative behavior and speech. Able to perform sacred rituals.
Yamya sattva	Free from mean and conflicting desires and acts. Having initiative, excellent memory, and leadership. Free from emotional binds, hatred, ignorance, and envy. The capacity for timely action.
Varuna sattva	Free from mean acts. Exhibition of emotions in proper place. Observance of religious rites.
Kabera sattva	Courage, patience, and hatred of impure thoughts. Liking for virtuous acts and purity. Pleasure in recreation.
Gandharva sattva	Possession of wealth, attendants, and luxuries. Expertise in poetry, stories, and epics. Fondness for dancing, singing, and music. Takes pleasure in perfumes, garlands, and flowers. Full of passion.

Sattvika individuals are generally noble and spiritually orientated.

They are not at all ostentatious in clothes or behavior.

Gastric problems are typical pitta–kapha complaints.

RIGHT *Giselle is a compassionate and selfless woman. She works hard to help others without desire for personal gain.*

SATTVIKA CHARACTERISTICS

Sattvika individuals are generally noble and spiritual in character. Their nature is determined not by body type alone but also their star constellation (*see* Astrology in Chapter Seven). In general, sattvika individuals will have an element of kapha in their constitutions, whether as the dominant dosha or along with the other doshas. Sattvika individuals belong to the following lunar signs:

Aswini	Anuradha	Hasta
Mrigasiras	Punarvasa	Pushya
Revati	Swati	Thiruvonam

The combinations of doshas would be:

kapha–pitta   pitta–kapha

kapha–vata   vata–kapha

CASE STUDY

Giselle is a typical sattvika person. The one very important characteristic of a sattvika person is their inability to lie. They are completely truthful in behavior. They are oriented toward work and compassion. Their main weaknesses are a fierce pride and a lack of humility.

Giselle works very hard as a medical doctor in London. She is heavily involved in local community activities. She is a member of a serious meditation group and spends at least an hour a day in meditation. She is not motivated by money or materialistic pursuits.

Her pitta–kapha character makes her irritable, but the kapha calms her and makes her forgiving and loving. She cannot lie, even to save her own life. Her pride does, however, make it difficult for her to accept the teaching of even the most venerable teacher.

She tends to suffer from the typical pitta–kapha complaints, including gastric problems and ovarian cysts.

Rajasika Individuals

The rajasika type of individual has a more wrathful disposition and has six subtypes based on the characteristic "antigodly" entities.

RAJASIKA SUBTYPES

SUBTYPES	QUALITIES
Asura	Indulgence in self-praise. Bravery, cruelty, envy, and ruthlessness. Terrifying appearance. Likes physical and verbal disguise.
Raksasa	Excessive sleep and indolence. Envious disposition. Constant anger, intolerance, and cruel behavior. Gluttonous habits.
Paisala	Unclean habits. Cowardly, with a terrifying disposition. Gluttonous habits. Fondness for opposite sex. Abnormal diet and regimen.
Sarpa	Sharp reactions. Excessive indolence. Frequent fearful disposition. Brave or cowardly attitude, depending on situation.
Praita	Excessive desire for food. Envious character. Excessive greediness and actions without discrimination.
Sakuna	Full of passion. Unsteadiness, ruthlessness, and excessive appetite for food.

CASE STUDY

James is a typical Rajasika person. He works hard some of the time but likes to take it easy when not pushed by his boss or necessity. He is quite willing to tell a few lies to get himself out of trouble but will not be totally dishonest or get somebody else into trouble or harm them by his actions.

He is alert to business opportunities and is a good marketing man. He has an excellent ability to perceive the strengths or weaknesses of other people and is very sensitive to human frailties.

As a pitta–vata individual, James is emotionally insecure and continually seeks relationships wherein he can replicate a maternal pattern of unconditional love before he is able to commit himself. He does not forgive people easily.

As a pitta–vata individual, his biggest physical problem is severe skin eruptions and irritable bowels.

RIGHT *Rajasika people are action-orientated and worldly. They make good executives and managers.*

RAJASIKA CHARACTERISTICS

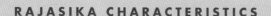

Rajasika individuals are very human in their character and their approach to life. They are intellectually oriented but vulnerable to the weaknesses and temptations of life. Like the other types, their nature is not determined simply by the body constitution but also by their lunar sign. Rajasika individuals are either pitta-dominated or have an element of pitta in their personality. Rajasika individuals belong to the following lunar signs:

Aridra	Bharan	Poorvabhadra
Poorvaphalguni	Poorvashada	Rohini
Uttara	Uttarabhadra	Uttrashada

Their dosha combinations would be:

pitta–kapha	kapha–pitta
pitta–vata	vata–pitta

Tamasika Individuals

TAMASIKA SUBTYPES

SUBTYPES	QUALITIES
Pasava	Lack of intelligence. Forbidding disposition. Envious nature. Excessive sexual indulgence and sleep.
Matsya	Unsteadiness, constant passion, and cowardice. Excessive desire for water intake.
Vanaspatya	Indolence. Excessive indulgence in food. Deficiency of intellectual faculties.

TAMASIKA CHARACTERISTICS

Tamasika individuals are the most down-to-earth of the three types. They are the "salt of the earth" and it is they who raise the fundamental questions of practical existence like food, shelter, sex, and entertainment when confronted by more individual, ethereal, or spiritual issues.

Tamasika individuals have a dominant element of vata in their constitution, though this is not the only factor that determines their character. They are born under tamasika or vata stars:

Aslesha   Chitra   Dhanishta   Jyeshta
Krittika   Makha   Moola   Satabisha
Visakha

The combination of doshas in the tamasika individual are:

vata–pitta   pitta–vata
vata–kapha   kapha–vata

CASE STUDY

François is a leading European painter. He has a vata–pitta constitution. He is slim and of medium height with light blue eyes. At 49 he still looks young for his age.

His vata–pitta constitution makes him restless but highly creative. He loves the sun but if it is too hot, he becomes irritable and breaks out in a rash.

Tamasika individuals are generally inclined toward an easy, relaxed life and dislike the routine of an office job or anything else that constrains them to a strict schedule.

Tamasika individuals are also liable to become dependent upon activities and objects that give them pleasure, like drink, cigarettes, and even drugs. They find it difficult to face any situation that can be tense or confrontational and, to that extent, try to avoid pain more than the other types.

François' combination of vata–pitta makes him a very intellectual painter with a powerful capacity to abstract the colors of life. His paintings are well-known for their precise composition and complex texture.

Yet, in his personal life he has found it difficult to form stable relationships. He has been married twice and has had a few unsuccessful relationships since then.

As a vata–pitta type he suffers from physical ailments unique to his mixture of personality traits and constitution. He has arthritis and rheumatic pains as well as a mild sexually transmitted disease through his slightly bohemian personal life.

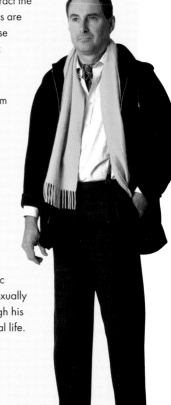

RIGHT *Tamasika individuals are unconventional and rebellious.*

The Prakrti ~
Our Individual Constitution

CONSTITUTIONAL FACTORS

Our prakrti is individual to each of us, and is known as our "constitution." The basic constitutional factors are the three doshas – vata, pitta, and kapha – and restoration of their dynamic balance regulates the life cycle and controls the entire body.

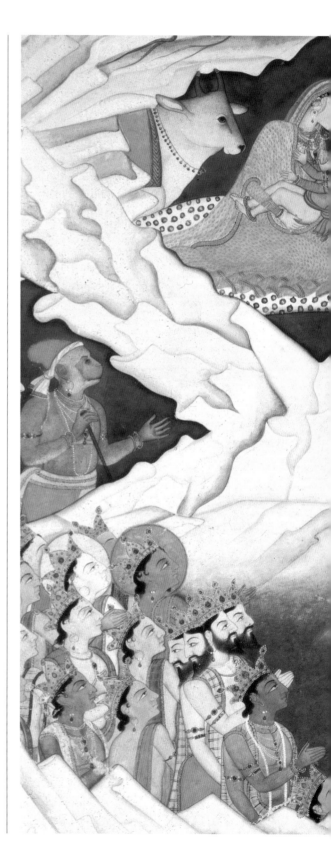

THE AYURVEDIC system of medicine lays special emphasis on your constitution or prakrti. Prakrti is determined not only by your dominant doshas, but by genetic factors, the condition of the uterus, nutrition, and lifestyle of the mother, and the five elements (panchamahabhutas) that make up the fetus.

Psychologists are now convinced that the experiences of the pregnant mother will influence the personality of her future child – and that these influences are even more vital and significant for a child than the events of infancy.

In this respect, prakrti has a genetic aspect, which is determined at the time of conception, as well as an acquired aspect determined by the mother's experiences.

Every individual has a different make-up and a different combination of the three doshas (*see* pages 46–59):

❀ In some people, vata is dominant (vatala prakrti)

❀ In some people, pitta is dominant (pittala prakrti)

❀ Other people are dominated by kapha (kaphaja prakrti)

Your prakrti, or constitution, determines your susceptibility to different diseases, the course and patterns that these diseases will follow, plus any complications that may arise and – of course – the prognosis of the disease.

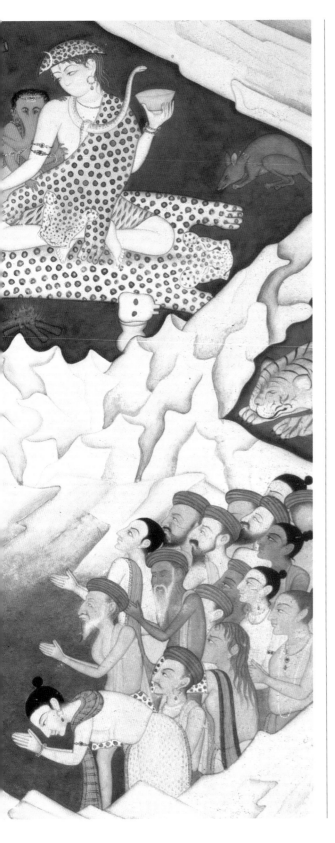

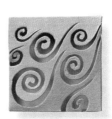

AIR

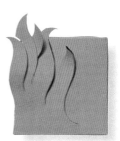

FIRE

LEFT *The Hindu god Shiva, with his consort, Parvati, on Mount Kailasa.*

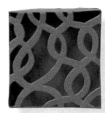

WATER

In addition to this, prakrti helps to explain your responses to treatments.

For all these reasons, prakrti is fundamental to Ayurvedic diagnosis and treatment, and is always first on the list of things for the Ayurvedic physician to examine. Depending on the predominant doshas, your prakrti can be divided into seven types:

- Vatika
- Paittika
- Kaphaja
- Vata paittika
- Vata kaphaja
- Pitta kaphaja
- Samdoshaja or Tridoshaja

The mixed types of prakrti (such as vata paittika, pitta kaphaja, and tridoshaja) will have mixed features according to the dominant doshas. Again, one or two doshas may dominate in one individual.

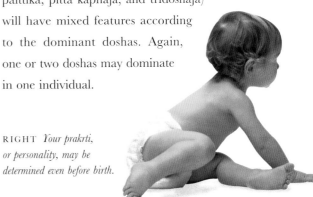

RIGHT *Your prakrti, or personality, may be determined even before birth.*

The Qualities of the Doshas

Kapha is oily, smooth, soft, firm, slow, dense, stable, heavy, cold, viscous, and clear. By virtue of these qualities, an individual having slesmala or kaphaja prakrti is endowed with excellence of strength, wealth, knowledge, energy, peace, and longevity.

Pitta is hot, sharp, liquid, sour, pungent, and of fleshy smell. By virtue of these qualities, the individual having pittala type of prakrti is endowed with moderate strength, moderate span of life, moderate spiritual and materialistic knowledge, wealth, and all accessories of life.

Vata is nonoily, light, mobile, swift, cold, rough, and nonslimy. Because of these qualities, an individual with vatala prakrti is endowed with average strength, average span of life, average procreation, average accessories of life, etc.

Individuals with constitutions dominated by the combination of two doshas reflect the qualities of those doshas. According to Charaka, a samdhatu type of individual who has all the doshas in a state of equilibrium is endowed with all the good qualities of all the three types of individuals.

The prakrti represents the individual constitution of each person, and since it involves both features of the mind and the body, an understanding of that prakrti will determine how to deal with disease on a holistic level. The practitioner considers the prakrti in order to determine the susceptibility of the individual to various diseases and how he or she might respond to the therapy prescribed. Assessment of the prakrti is essential for diagnosis, and no treatment will be prescribed without it.

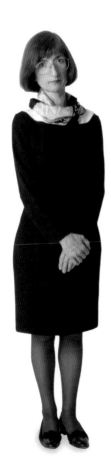 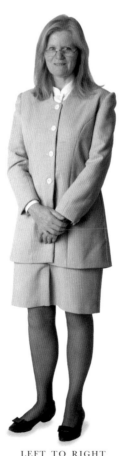 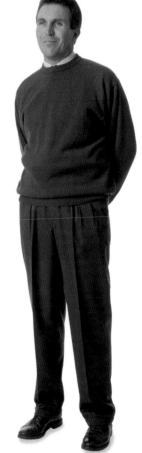

LEFT TO RIGHT
The friendly vata type, the cautious, shrewd pitta type, and the slow, affectionate kapha type.

CHARACTERISTICS OF PEOPLE WITH KAPHA PRAKRTI

ATTRIBUTES OF KAPHA	FEATURES MANIFESTED
Oily	Oiliness of organs, tissues, and skin.
Smooth	Smooth and soft skin.
Soft	Attractive appearance, soft and clear complexion.
Sweet	Increased sex drive, and good energy.
Firm	Large, firm, thick, and well-built joints. Firmness, compactness, and stability of the body.
Dense	Thick, broad, well-developed body. Plumpness and roundness.
Slow	Pulse is slow, deep, and swan-like.
Stable	Mentally logical and stable. Graceful and stable gait.
Heavy	Heavy, tending toward obesity.
Cold	Intolerant of cold and damp.
Viscous	Firmness and compactness of joints.
Clear	Deep, pleasant, clear, and resonant voice.

CHARACTERISTICS OF PEOPLE WITH VATA PRAKRTI

ATTRIBUTES OF VATA	FEATURES MANIFESTED
Lack of oiliness	Underdeveloped body, flat and depressed chest. Weak, low, and hoarse voice.
Light	Light movements. Irregular and erratic appetite. Thin, small, and cracking joints.
Mobile	Quick, short steps. Fast.
Abundance	Talkative. Frequent sex drive.
Swift	Quick in action. Pulse is rapid, thready, and snake-like.
Cold	Intolerant of cold, wind, and dry weather. Often inflicted with cold and shivering.
Rough	Hair is dry, coarse, and curly. Skin is rough, thin, cracked, and flaky.

CHARACTERISTICS OF PEOPLE WITH PITTA PRAKRTI

ATTRIBUTES OF PITTA	FEATURES MANIFESTED
Hot	Intolerant of heat and sun. Sweating with strong odor. Skin is warm, moist, with freckles, black moles, acne, etc. Early graying of hair and baldness. Warm hands and feet.
Sharp	Sharp appetite, strong digestive power, intake of large quantity of food and drinks. Sharp and high-pitched voice.
Liquid	Medium soft and loose joints and muscle. Abundance of sweat, urine, and feces.
Fleshy smell	Profuse strong odor from various parts of body – axilla, mouth, head, and body.
Pungent and sour taste	Liking for sweet, light, warm, pungent, and sour taste. Moderate sexual desire.

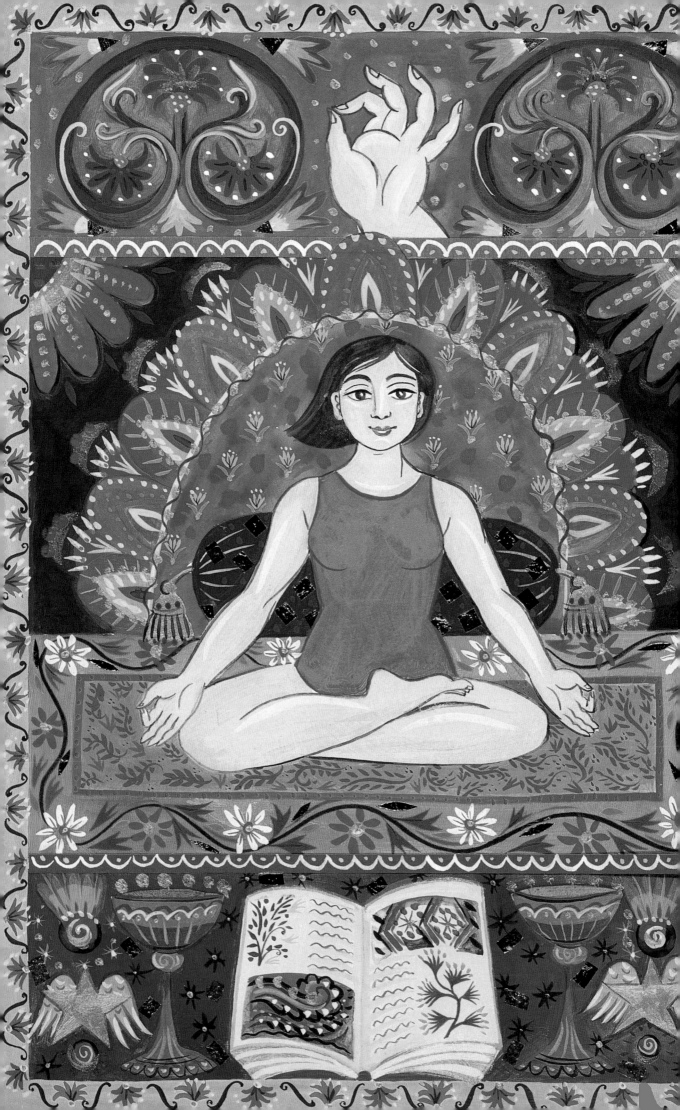

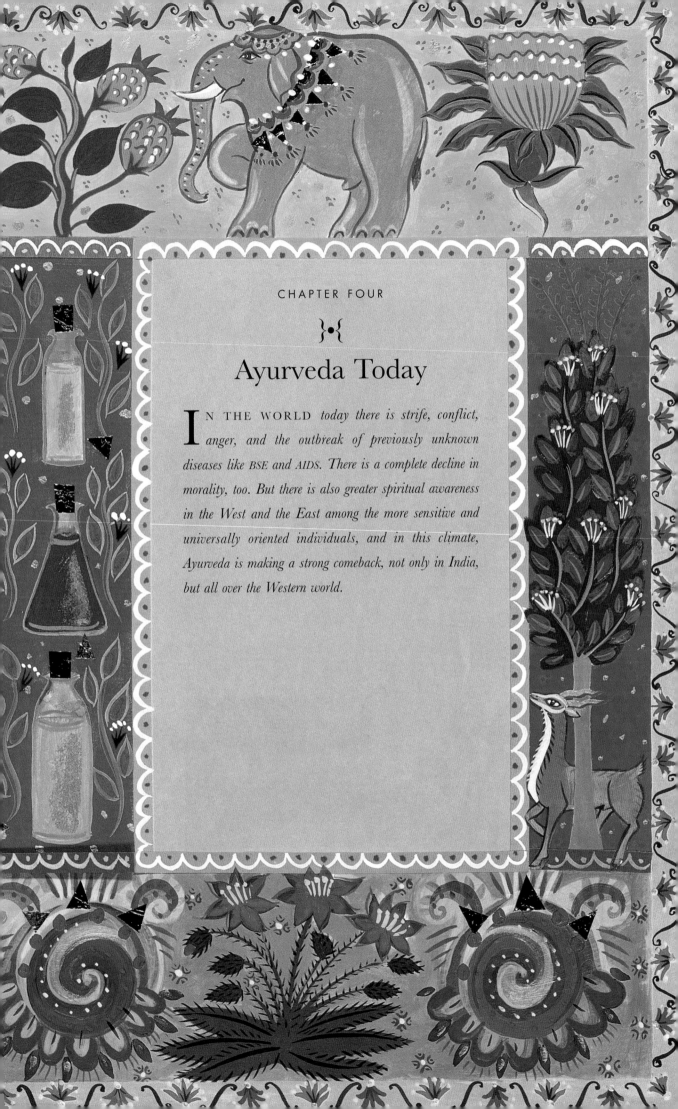

CHAPTER FOUR

⊱•⊰

Ayurveda Today

IN THE WORLD *today there is strife, conflict,
anger, and the outbreak of previously unknown
diseases like* BSE *and* AIDS. *There is a complete decline in
morality, too. But there is also greater spiritual awareness
in the West and the East among the more sensitive and
universally oriented individuals, and in this climate,
Ayurveda is making a strong comeback, not only in India,
but all over the Western world.*

Ayurveda in the West

TODAY, in the Western world, beset by strife, moral confusion, conflict, and disease, there is more need than ever for the kind of wisdom and vision that can save humanity from itself and restore harmony. There are positive signs that the time is right for Ayurveda in the West. Increasingly, people have come to understand the links between mind and body, and complementary therapies are in demand as never before.

There is also a new awareness of the oneness of creation, reflected in the growth of a strong green movement, a trend to vegetarianism, and an emphasis on eating healthier, organically grown wholefoods. There is also a sense of spiritual awakening in the West, and an interest in the religions and beliefs of people around the world.

Unfortunately, there is a habit in the West of referring to everything in decades, not centuries or yugas (Hindu ages). People say that this was the fashion in the 1960s, something else in the 1970s, and so on.

To those born in the East where the *Mahabharata*, (an epic of ancient India) which happened 4,000 years ago, is still retold to a newborn child in the family, the rise and fall of fads in the West is disconcerting as the tendency to trivialize, commercialize, and exploit even profound and sacred knowledge leads to the kind of amorality and confusion of values that is rampant in the West today.

Ayurveda, in this sense, is the latest "craze" to arrive in the West after yoga, transcendental meditation (TM), and levitation, not to mention the self-grown techniques like aromatherapy, Rolfing, the Alexander technique, and a host of others. However, the profound history, tradition, and spirit of Ayurveda set it aside from faddish new theories.

To preserve Ayurveda in its true form, it is necessary to prevent the dilution and distortion that have happened in the case of meditation, yoga, and such esoteric practices as Tantra and Vajrayana Buddhism. The Western need to adapt all spiritual disciplines to appease consumer demand at any cost is a mutagen that Ayurveda will have to try hard to resist.

There is, however, a very serious incongruity between the extensive "hype" that Ayurveda has recently received in the West and the absence of fully qualified Ayurvedic practitioners and authentic Ayurvedic medicines in the same countries.

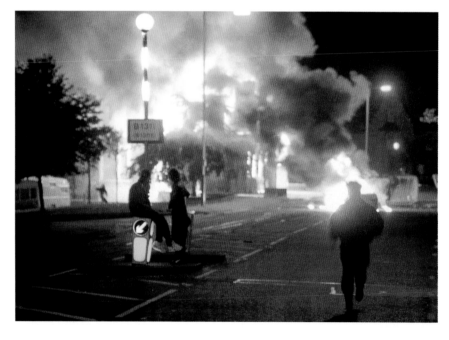

LEFT *Under the stresses and strains of modern urban living, tension sometimes breaks out in aggressive forms.*

DEEP ROOTS

Ayurveda has survived in India for over 5,000 years, in spite of a century-long ban by the British. It survives because it has deep roots within Hindu philosophy and because it succeeds as a natural and safe treatment for otherwise incurable ailments.

A SERIOUS SHORTAGE

There is a very serious incongruity between the extensive hype that Ayurveda has recently received in the West and the absence of fully qualified Ayurvedic practitioners and authentic Ayurvedic medicines in those same countries.

KARMA IS A SLOW VIRUS

As we write this book, a university scientist is describing on the television news the possibility of using specially developed pigs' organs, particularly hearts, for transplant into human beings. There is no serious debate or objection being raised to this transgression of the natural order. The concerned scientist states confidently that there is no known possibility of pig viruses entering the human chain!

It is ironic that this is followed by the news of further culling of British cows affected by the BSE virus. The scientific world does not seem to accept the recent history of mutation of scrapie into BSE in cows and Creutzfeld-Jacob's Disease in humans. The following stanza comes from a poem written by the author 15 years ago, entitled "Karma is a Slow Virus."

> Like a mole, an unpleasant wart
> Karma is a slow virus
> encrusted on the soul of man.
> "Kuru" and "Creutzfeld-Jacob"
> may take twenty years to manifest but
> Karma has no life-expectancy,
> taking lifetimes before it dawns as a dark
> terror in the afternoon of a life
> that didn't seem to deserve such sorrow.

RIGHT *The natural order of the world should be respected, or we may be subjected to more new diseases, such as the BSE virus now found in British cows.*

Scientists do not seem to understand that even their inventions are governed by the laws of karma, the inescapable law of action and reaction that governs the manifested universe.

Ayurveda re-establishes the primacy of the natural cycle of the cosmos. Its correct practice has the capacity to cleanse and strengthen not merely the human species but even the earth herself. This is what the sacred mantra of Dhanwantari reveals and what the West and the world need today: a simpler and quieter life, a more reflective and introspective life governed by the rhythm of nature and the universe. Ayurveda is the barometer to measure and interpret these rhythms.

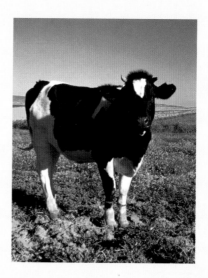

Ayurveda in India

MOST OLD disciplines die or get distorted due to the passage of time. New forms of meditation, yogic exercises, and even religious rituals show how social and economic change create variations of old practices.

On the other hand, a number of spiritual and religious practices have been forgotten or lost, like the daily fire ritual that was once a part of the upbringing of most Hindus. Even the meditation on the Gayatri Mantra that was once a must for every Brahmin (a person of the highest caste of Hindu society) is now hardly uttered by modern Indian youth.

Fortunately Ayurveda, even though it is older than most religious practices of India, has maintained its popularity there and, in fact, has made a major comeback, despite a number of attempts to suppress it during the colonial days in order to promote Western medicine.

During the 150-odd years of British rule in India, most upper- and upper middle-class Indian families sent one of their children to study Western medicine and to become a physician. Today India has the second-largest number of trained physicians in the world, and Indian physicians in large numbers support the medical systems in the U.K. and the U.S.A.

However, in this period Ayurveda became a second-class option, and the intellectual elite was creamed off by Western medicine. Yet the village poor still turned to Ayurveda, because few Western-trained doctors were prepared to go and work in the villages. In spite of their wealth affording them the possibility of using Western medicine, the aristocrats and the

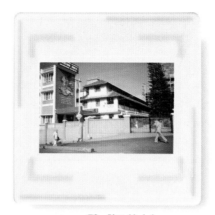

ABOVE *The Kottakkal Arya Vaidya Sala in Kerala, India, founded by P. S. Warrier.*

maharajas also supported Ayurveda. The Sanskrit scholars, the spiritually minded and orthodox Hindus also continued to follow Ayurveda.

A few institutions, like the Kottakkal Arya Vaidya Sala, the Arya Vaidya Pharmacy in Coimbatore, and the Benares Hindu University kept alive the noble traditions of Ayurveda in their pristine form. Ayurvedic hospitals became the last refuge for rejects from the Western medical system who could not be cured of chronic long-term ailments like asthma, rheumatoid arthritis, and skin diseases.

Today, there has been a sea change. Ayurveda is now a thriving science, and more than 500 new Ayurvedic companies and Ayurvedic hospitals have been set up in India in the last 10 years alone. Orthodox physicians and Ayurvedic physicians now work alongside one another.

AYURVEDA IN THE WEST

Spiritual and Ecological Movements

✤ **Strong green movement**

✤ **Spiritual philosophies of Ayurveda**

✤ **Trend toward vegetarianism**

✤ **Increasing antipathy toward modern drugs, especially by long-term sufferers**

✤ **Well publicized dangers of certain drugs, e.g. Opren, anti-inflammatories, tranquilizers**

✤ **Paradigm shift toward holistic and systems approach in the scientific community**

✤ **Increasing acceptance of links between mind and body**

✤ **Growth of alternative therapies**

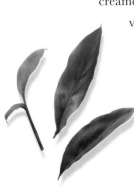

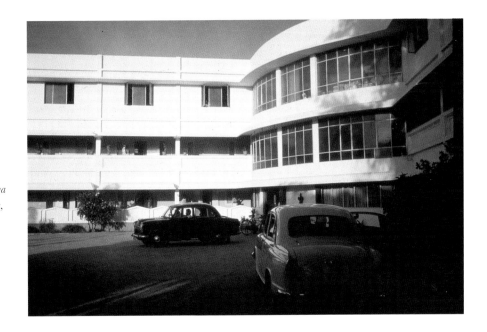

RIGHT *The Arya Vaidya Pharmacy in Tamil Nadu, a leading Ayurvedic hospital founded by P. V. Rama Warrier.*

BELOW *An old-fashioned Ayurvedic medical shop in India.*

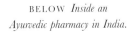

BELOW *Inside an Ayurvedic pharmacy in India.*

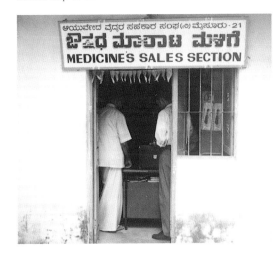

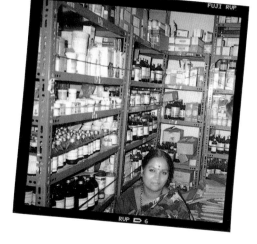

BELOW RIGHT *A modern Ayurvedic laboratory in India.*

RIGHT *People of all social classes visit Ayurvedic physicians for treatment.*

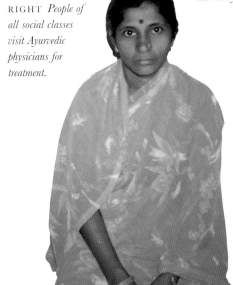

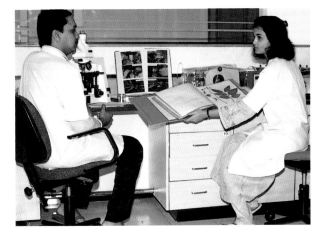

Ayurveda and Modern Medicine Working Together

AYURVEDA has cures for most, if not all, chronic ailments. By following the precepts of Ayurveda, most illnesses (even the common cold) can be avoided. However, there are a number of cases where Ayurvedic medicine cannot have immediate effect and the patient could develop serious or fatal complications. These include:

- Acute infections and illnesses (cholera, typhoid, smallpox, acute meningitis, viral fevers)
- Emergency surgical cases including all accidents (e.g., appendicitis, hernia, major wounds, intestinal obstruction)
- Myocardial infarction (heart attacks)

Even in such cases, however, Ayurveda has been effectively used in India as an adjunct to modern surgical treatment and medicine.

For example, postoperative recovery in accident victims can be much quicker if Ayurvedic massage is used with physiotherapy. Ayurvedic oils such as:

- Sahacharadia thailam
- Maharajaprasarini thailam
- Gandha thailam
- Kottamchukkadi thailam

have a magical effect on the speed of recovery of sports injuries and postsurgical cases.

A number of Ayurvedic medicines are also used by Western trained physicians in India as adjuncts to Western medicine. Preparations containing guggul *(commiphora mukul)* are often used with antibiotics as anti-infectives and anti-inflammatories to reduce the dosage and length of treatment by powerful antibiotics with serious side effects.

The conventional Ayurvedic physician will frown and disapprove of such mixed therapies, but in the hectic modern world, where few patients follow the Ayurvedic way of life, there are conditions that require emergency treatment where powerful modern medicine has a role to play.

Such conditions test the wisdom, experience, and training of Ayurvedic physicians, but there have been, and still are, legendary Ayurvedic physicians to whom even acute emergencies with surgical needs do not pose a problem. Such physicians, however, move from the domain of the average physician to highly evolved spiritual beings who have transcended the domain of ordinary existence and become healers with an almost divine touch.

BELOW *Physiotherapy forms an important part of Western medical treatment for injuries.*

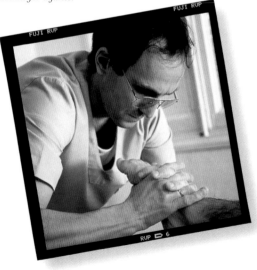

BELOW *Intensive Ayurvedic massage can accelerate the healing process and speed recovery.*

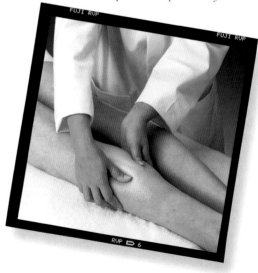

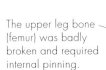

Robert's upper body was weakened by prolonged inactivity, but soon recovered with appropriate exercise.

The upper leg bone (femur) was badly broken and required internal pinning.

There was extensive damage to the cartilage and ligaments of the knee joint, requiring complex surgery.

CASE STUDY

Robert, a man in his mid 40s, had to undergo an emergency operation after sustaining serious leg injuries in a major motor accident. His knee and thigh had been crushed in the accident. The extent of his injuries and the number of pins that had to be used internally suggested that there would be a long period of physiotherapy, possibly up to one year. It was thought that further operations might even be necessary. However, as soon as his scars had healed, Robert was given continuous Ayurvedic massage and he was able to shorten his recovery period to four months instead of the anticipated year.

The left leg was forced to work harder while the right leg was immobilized, but massage and physiotherapy combined to redress the muscular imbalance.

LEFT *Injured in a car crash, this patient underwent a very beneficial combination of Western and Ayurvedic treatment, leading to a full and speedy recovery.*

Applying Ayurveda to Our Daily Lives

AYURVEDA is useful for the treatment of almost any condition, as it addresses the body as a whole. The following conditions in particular should respond to treatment:

- Digestive complaints such as irritable bowel syndrome, constipation, and indigestion
- Eczema
- Skin problems
- Insomnia
- Allergies
- Back pain
- Bronchitis
- Eye disease
- Colds
- Anxiety
- Sinusitis
- Rheumatoid arthritis
- High blood pressure
- Circulatory problems
- Headaches and migraines
- Paralysis (partial and complete)
- Irritability and emotional stress

Ayurveda will keep the immune system strong and capable of fighting off infection, and enable it to address chronic disorders from within.

Ayurvedic lifestyle, diagnosis, and treatment, are described in Chapters Five, Six, and Seven.

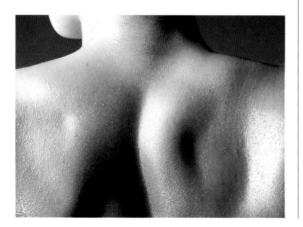

HOW DO I FIND A GOOD AYURVEDIC PHYSICIAN?

To practice Ayurvedic medicine takes just as much dedication and training as to become a qualified physician in the West – if not more. Like a Western medic, the Ayurvedic physician has to be expert in anatomy, physiology, botany, and pharmacology, but must also have a good knowledge of Sanskrit and Indian philosophy, religion, and yoga. And there are the different disciplines of Ayurveda to master – such as diet and lifestyle – together with astrology and the interpretation of events and omens symbolizing karmic patterns. Even the most highly trained and expert person will not be a good Ayurvedic physician without the right attitudes. Compassion, understanding of karma, and motivation that is free from greed are at the heart of Ayurveda. Unfortunately, there is a serious shortage of qualified Ayurvedic practitioners and authentic medicines to meet the current demand in the West. We estimate that there are fewer than 100 qualified Ayurvedic practitioners in the U.K. and fewer than 50 in the U.S.A.

In the hands of a qualified practitioner (*see* opposite page), Ayurvedic medicine is completely safe for people of all ages and levels of health. Some treatments may be unsuitable for pregnant women and children, or for very ill or frail adults, but treatment is always tailored to the individual, and a qualified practitioner would never recommend anything that is contraindicated.

LEFT *Troublesome back pain often responds positively to Ayurvedic treatment, especially with massage.*

ABOVE *Clinical trials have shown that eczema can be successfully treated with Ayurvedic medicines.*

An Ayurvedic practitioner should:

- Be qualified from a university in India or Sri Lanka
- Have completed a five-year degree course
- Have completed a one-year internship in an Ayurvedic hospital.

Please ensure that your practitioner has the above qualifications before undergoing treatment and, if nothing else, that he is a properly licensed healthcare professional.

The pattern of Ayurvedic practice in the West has followed the settlement of Indian people in the West and this has focused mainly in the U.K. and in the U.S.A.

A leading fully qualified Western practitioner of Ayurveda is Dr. Robert Svobodo who lives in the U.S.A and has written a number of excellent books on the subject. It is our contention that to practice Ayurveda anywhere in the world the practitioner should have undergone a full five-year university degree in Ayurveda, unless they are already qualified doctors and nurses, in which case a reduction in the number of years required to three could be considered.

AYURVEDIC PRACTITIONERS

Our estimated numbers of fully qualified Ayurvedic practitioners who are permanently resident in Europe and the USA are as follows:

USA
Less than
50

Europe
Less than
200

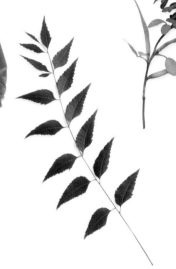

ABOVE AND LEFT Trigonella foenum gracecum *and* Azadirachta indica, *both used in Ayurvedic medicine.*

LEFT *All Ayurvedic physicians should undergo a five-year degree in Ayurveda plus a year of hospital training.*

FAR LEFT *Mortar and pestle used for grinding plants and other ingredients into a fine powder.*

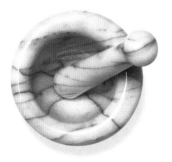

Ayurveda: A Powerful Science

WITHOUT THE extensive knowledge that is required to become an Ayurvedic practitioner, it is dangerous to practice Ayurvedic medicine, or even to counsel patients using Ayurvedic disciplines. Ayurveda is a powerful science, and if practiced by unskilled hands it could pose a serious risk to health and well-being. Many Ayurvedic medicines are intended for use only by physicians with a thorough knowledge of their effects and of the "pathya," or the changes in diet and lifestyle, that are necessary for them to work to best effect. Without this regimen, and the wide knowledge of the possible pitfalls, the treatment could be at best ineffective and, at worst, dangerous.

You would never agree to having an operation performed by a Western physician with only a few months of training. In the same way, you should steer clear of any Ayurvedic practitioner who has not had sufficient training and experience.

There are four main issues that should be considered concerning the new trend toward untrained Ayurvedic practitioners jumping on the complementary-medicine bandwagon.

❀ There is a serious danger to patients, both on a spiritual and physical level. Incorrect treatment can cause problems.

❀ There is a danger to the science of Ayurveda and its reputation. If incorrect treatment creates a bad reputation for Ayurveda, then there will be a government backlash leading to legislative restrictions in Western countries. This has already happened in the case of some Ayurvedic medicines that have been misused. This will prevent Ayurveda from reaching the public who deserve its help.

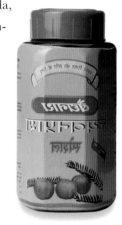

❀ Developing countries, such as India and Sri Lanka, have thousands of genuine practitioners who are capable of offering skilled treatment; many of them are forced to practice covertly in the West while charlatans are able to treat people quite openly.

❀ Ayurvedic products that are unproven and often inferior substitutes are available to the general public. They claim to have similar effects to genuine Ayurvedic products, again undermining the reputation of the real thing, and "spoiling" the market for products that are actually effective.

❀ There is also the question of the unfair and invisible trade barriers on the import and sale of authentic Ayurvedic products with the result that untested, unproven, and often inferior substitutes are used claiming similar effect to genuine Ayurvedic products. For the economic and developmental issues of these barriers, see page 82.

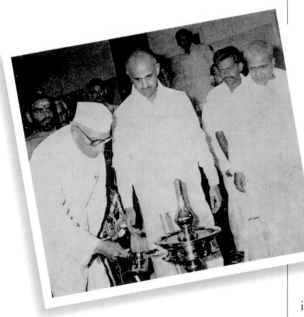

ABOVE *The former Prime Minister of India, Mr. Desai, opening a new wing of the Arya Vaidya Pharmacy Hospital.*

ABOVE RIGHT *The Ayurvedic tonic for general health and bronchial complaints, chyavana prasam.*

CHAKRA AND MARMA THERAPY

Two potentially dangerous concepts that have been ill-used by untrained practitioners are:

✤ Opening the chakras

✤ Marma therapy

Any responsible Ayurvedic physician or spiritual teacher will clearly warn the layman, or even an advanced seeker or practitioner, against indulging in either of these practices.

However, these days, a number of alternative practitioners do offer both. Books are written on how to open one's chakras, and a modern dance artiste even performed a "chakra opening" dance, combined with Ayurvedic massage, on stage in London.

Opening the chakras should not be practiced at all, other than under a spiritual guide. It is extremely dangerous and can drive people insane. Even the idea of simply attempting to open the chakras is a nonsense, because it is a process of spiritual evolution that can take many lifetimes.

Chakras are a part of spiritual development, not of Ayurveda. To progress spiritually from one chakra to the next, according to any teacher, takes many lifetimes. Anyone who attempts to "open" them by focusing on them is inviting trouble for themselves. At our clinics we have had a number of cases of Westerners who have learned how to "open" chakras from books, and got themselves into a state of serious mental and psychological confusion, if not derangement. Chakras are best left well alone!

Marma therapy poses an even more immediate threat. Marma therapy should be practiced only by Ayurvedic physicians who have had a number of years of experience under marma experts. While the correct use of marma techniques can cure illnesses effectively, their wrong use can be fatal. Touching specific marmas with incorrect force or at the wrong time can even cause death.

Marma therapy is a very complex Ayurvedic treatment and requires vast experience, in terms of both training and theory, as well as years of practice. An inexperienced practitioner could cause serious or fatal damage to a patient undergoing marma therapy. Please steer clear of anyone who offers you this form of therapy unless they have a full Ayurvedic degree and at least ten years of practice.

Those who are true spiritual masters or great marma experts will never talk lightly about these subjects. Please treat anyone who speaks or writes easily about these two subjects with a considerable degree of scepticism.

LEFT *Marma therapy and chakra "openings" should not be practiced by untrained or lay people.*

The Invisible Trade Barriers to Ayurvedic Products

THE U.S.A. AND EUROPE have the largest share of the herbal product market, and with strict legislation against new products entering the market, there is very little opportunity for authentic Ayurvedic products to be sold in the West. Many of the herbal products that are sold are inefficient, with no clinical or toxicological evidence to support them, yet the licensing system operates on the criterion that native products should be given priority. It is, therefore, very difficult for the spread of genuine Ayurvedic products to make their way into Western stores and, because Ayurvedic practitioners present competition to native herbalists, there is little support from the industry. Perhaps one of the most important points about this problem is that if Indian and Chinese herbal medical products were allowed to be sold freely in Western countries, and Ayurvedic and Chinese practitioners were allowed to practice without restrictions (but subject to status regulations) to meet public demand for genuine products, there could be a significant economic impact upon these developing countries from export resources.

The most effective way to spread Ayurveda in the West in a way that benefits the people needing treatment and guidance is to:

❋ Ensure that legislation allows Ayurvedic physicians from India to practice freely in the West,

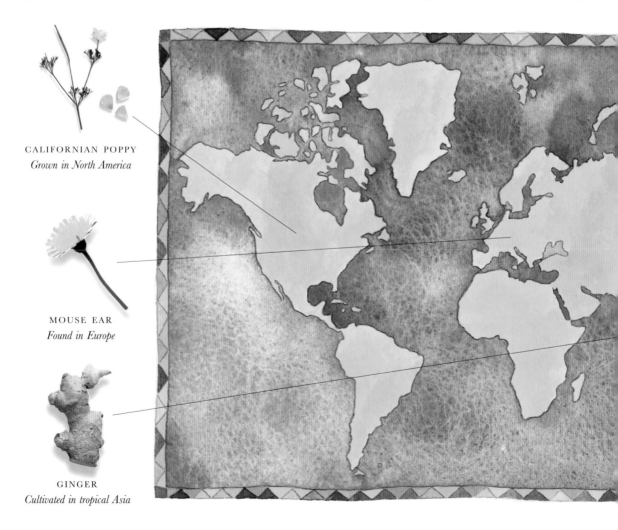

CALIFORNIAN POPPY
Grown in North America

MOUSE EAR
Found in Europe

GINGER
Cultivated in tropical Asia

subject to their qualifications and residential status being acceptable to the accrediting universities and governments of the host countries.

❖ Allow the establishment and recognition of accreditation centers in each country to help the process of accreditation by bodies qualified to do so.

❖ Allow the free import and sale of quality Ayurvedic products from established manufacturers and allow them to advertise and promote their products, subject to the same accreditation guidelines.

❖ Assist in the establishment of Ayurvedic colleges and hospitals so that local people can be fully trained to degree level in Ayurveda.

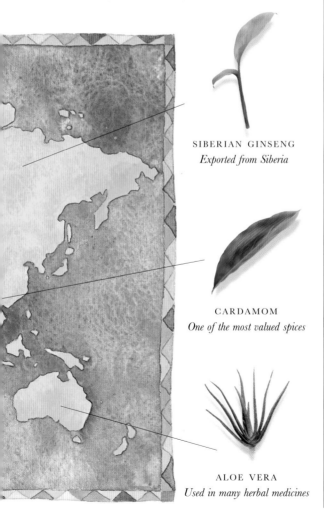

SIBERIAN GINSENG
Exported from Siberia

CARDAMOM
One of the most valued spices

ALOE VERA
Used in many herbal medicines

HERBAL AND AYURVEDIC SALES

Ayurvedic Sales 1996

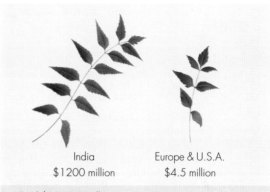

| India $1200 million | Europe & U.S.A. $4.5 million |

Total $1204.5 million

Herbal Sales

Country	Herbal Medicine Market Size ($m)	Consumption Per Capita (p.a. $)
Germany	2,100.0	27.03
France	174.0	3.075
United Kingdom	132.0	2.295
Italy	123.0	2.13
Denmark	93.0	18.24
Spain	45.0	1.17
Belgium	39.0	3.945
Netherlands	37.5	2.505
Portugal	18.0	1.815
Ireland	5.4	1.545
Greece	1.05	0.105
Luxembourg	0.9	2.25
Total	2,768.85	8.115*
Other E.E.C.	75.0	N.A.
U.S.A.	1350.0	5.55
Canada	75.0	2.55

Total   over $4,200 million

* weighted by population size in order to give the average per capita spending per annum.

Ayurvedic sales, it may be seen, do not form even 1% of the herbal sales in the West, even though a number of herbal ingredients from India are imported.

Many Active Ingredients

There is no single active ingredient in Ayurvedic medicines. Ayurvedic treatments and remedies are synergistic – so that each ingredient supports the activity of other ingredients.

Unfortunately, most Western medical control agencies (such as the Food and Drug Administration and the Medicines Control Agency insist on single-ingredient products. In contrast, most Ayurvedic medicines contain between 5 and 25 ingredients, including herbs and minerals, and for effective treatment these must be formulated in the correct combination to balance the doshas that are being treated.

VASAK
Adhatoda vasica

Liv 52 is one of the most popular Ayurvedic medicines for hepatitis and liver problems, and it has proved, in over two hundred studies, to be effective in the treatment and cure of hepatitis A and B, as well as the new non-A, non-B category. Liv 52 contains eight ingredients – *Capparis spinosa, Cichorium intybus, Mandur bhasma, Solanum nigrum, Terminalia arjuna, Cassia occidentalis, Achillea millefolium, and Tamaris.*

Many Ayurvedic medicines contain a far larger number and range of substances, as the lists of active ingredients for three other medicines shown on these pages indicate.

PIPPALI
Piper longum

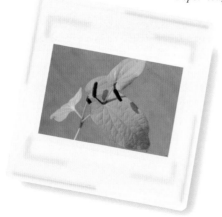

BRONCHITIS, COUGHS, EMPHYSEMA
Vasarishtam – Composition

Sanskrit Name	Latin/English Name
Vasak	*Adhatoda vasica*
Jal	Water
Gur	Jaggery
Dhaipushpa	*Woodfordia floribunda*
Dalchini	*Cinnamomum zeylanicum*
Ela	*Elettaria cardamomum*
Tejpatra	*Cinnamomum iners*
Nagkeshar	*Mesua ferrea*
Kankol	*Piper cubeb*
Sunthi	*Zingiber officinale*
Kalamarich	*Piper nigrum*
Pippali	*Piper longum*
Sugandh Bala	*Valeriana officinalis*

CYSTITIS, URINARY INFECTIONS
Chandanasava – Composition

Sanskrit Name	Latin/English Name
Chandan (Swet)	*Santalum album*
Sugandha Bala	*Valerina officinalis*
Mustak	*Cyperus rotundus*
Neel Kamal	*Nelumbium spiciosum*
Priyangu	*Callicarpa macrophylla*
Padmakasth	*Prunus puddum*
Lodhra Chhal	*Symplocos racemosa*
Manjishtha	*Rubia cordifolia*
Raktachandan	*Pterocarpus santalinus*
Patha	*Cissampelos pareira*
Chirayata	*Swertia chirata*
Batchhal	*Ficus bengalensis*
Pippal Chhal	*Ficus relegiosa*
Sathi	*Salvia plebela*
Pitta papra	*Fumaria offinalis*
Mulethi	*Glycyrrhiza glabra*
Rasna	*Vanda roxburghii*
Patol Patra	*Trico santhes dioica*
Kanchnar Chhal	*Bauchinia tomentosa*
Amrachhal	*Mangifera indica*
Moch Ras	*Bombax malabarica*
Dhataki Pushpa	*Woodfordia floribunda*
Draksha	*Vitis vinifera*
Jal	Water
Sharkara	Sugar
Gur	Jaggery

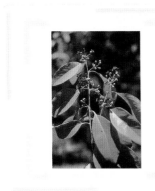

CHANDAN
Santalum album

ARTHRITIS, RHEUMATISM

Maha Yograj Guggul – Composition

Sanskrit Name	Latin/English Name
Shunthi	*Zingiber officinale*
Pippali mool	*Piper longum* root
Pippali	*Piper longum*
Chabya	*Piper chaba*
Chitrak mool	*Plumbago zeylanica*
Shuddha hing	Pure *Asafoetida*
Ajmoda	*Apium graveolens*
Sarson	*Brassica alba*
Jeera (Shwet)	*Cumminum cyminum*
Jeera (Kala)	*Nigella sativa*
Renuka	*Piper auranticum*
Patha	*Cissampelos pareira*
Vidanga	*Embelia ribes*
Gaj pippali	*Plantago amplexicaulis*
Kutaki	*Picrorrhiza kurrooa*
Atibisha	*Aconitum heterophyllum*
Bharangi	*Clerodendrum serratum*
Bach	*Acorus calamus*
Murwa	*Sansevieria roxburghiana*
Haritaki	*Terminalia chebula*
Amla	*Emblica officinalis*
Bahera	*Terminalia belerica*
Shuddha guggul	Pure *Commiphora mukul*
Banga bhasma	*Stannum* calcined
Ropya bhasma	Silver calcined
Nag bhasma	Lead calcined
Lauh bhasma	Iron calcined
Abhrak bhasma	Mica calcined
Mandoor bhasma	Ironrust calcined

SCIENTIFIC VALIDATION OF AYURVEDA

It is not time alone that has proven the efficacy of Ayurvedic medicines and treatment. There have been over fifty thousand major scientific research projects into Ayurvedic products, all of these led by qualified medical personnel and P.h.D.s in pharmacology. A number of these projects include double-blind trials on Ayurvedic products.

The Herbal Medical Database in London lists over twenty thousand trials on Ayurvedic products conducted in India and the West. These include trials on Ayurvedic compound medicines with a number of ingredients, as well as on Ayurvedic herbs.

The Herbal Medical Database was created over ten years ago and now has over one hundred thousand entries on herbal medicine with clinical and toxicological trials on European, American, Chinese, and Ayurvedic herbal medicines and plants. This company also publishes market research reports on a syndicated basis as well as for individual clients. The Database is particularly strong in Ayurvedic medicines, which are now gaining ground across the world and particularly in the United States.

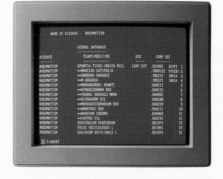

ABOVE *The computer of the Herbal Medical Database showing the typical medicinal plants used for rheumatism.*

Clinical Trials

Clinical trials are a necessity for any prescribed pharmaceutical product and for any product that makes a medical claim. They are the "scientific" method of verifying the efficacy of a particular medicine or treatment system, and they fulfill two main purposes.

First, clinical trials establish the successful repeatability of the treatment for other patients. Second, they rule out the possibility that a cure is due to the placebo, or psychosomatic, effect.

Since Ayurveda takes this effect strongly into consideration, and since Ayurvedic theory holds that each patient is unique, the clinical trial system is not necessarily best equipped to test the Ayurvedic system of medicine. Nonetheless, a number of Ayurvedic medicines have been tested for clinical efficacy through double-blind trials. These involve one or more physicians, and two groups of patients suffering from the same illness, with the same level of symptoms, and belonging to the same age group. Gender representation in each group is also similar.

The case histories of both groups of patients are carefully studied, and various tests are carried out. Medications being given to the patients at a particular time are carefully noted, and are then either withdrawn or made uniform throughout the two groups if the drugs are life-supporting.

The medicine to be tested is then administered to one group of patients, and the other group is given a placebo that looks exactly the same but has no effect at all. Neither the patients nor the doctors treating them are aware who is receiving the placebo and who is taking the real medicine.

The patients are carefully monitored during the tests to detect any sign of progress or deterioration. At the end of the test, the results are analyzed and tabulated, and a research paper is published.

Clinical trials on Ayurvedic medicine, including double-blind trials, are given in this section.

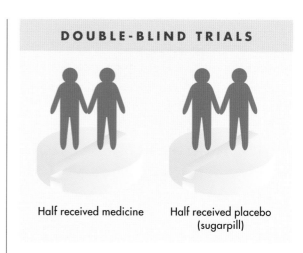

DOUBLE-BLIND TRIALS

Half received medicine

Half received placebo (sugarpill)

In the case of Ayurvedic treatment, as opposed to a simple Ayurvedic medicine, double-blind trials are virtually impossible. This is because Ayurvedic treatment consists of far more than simply giving pills to a patient. It involves a number of therapies in addition to the medication, including:

- Dietary regulation and changes
- Lifestyle changes
- Panchakarma (detoxification)
- Rejuvenation and rebalancing
- Yoga therapy
- Spiritual advice

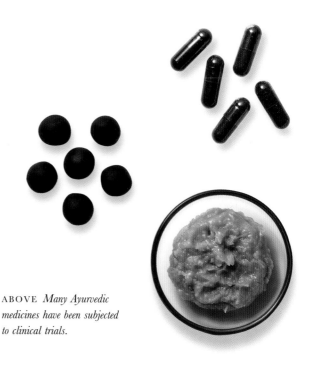

ABOVE *Many Ayurvedic medicines have been subjected to clinical trials.*

If one were asked to place a percentage on the importance of medicine in treatment, one would hesitate to put it above 60 percent. Medicine plus panchakarma will form 80 percent of the treatment.

In such a system, a double-blind trial of the whole treatment system is impossible, because one cannot give panchakarma without the knowledge of the doctor or the patient, or while using a placebo.

With a seven-thousand-year record of successful treatment, Ayurveda has certainly stood the test of time, but there are also many thousands of medical studies that show that the Ayurvedic system of medicine can help to treat various diseases.

Here are some examples of trials on herbal products commonly used in Ayurvedic treatment, including the most important Ayurvedic medicine, guggul, used extensively for rheumatoid arthritis, osteoarthritis, and other major complications.

HERBAL PRODUCT TRIAL 2

❖ TITLE *Effect of guggul (Commiphora mukul) on serum lipids in obese hypercholestremic cases*

❖ SOURCE *J Ass Physns Ind, 1978, 26(5), 3670373*

❖ AUTHORS *Kuppurjan, K., Rajagopalan, S.*

❖ Effect of oral administration of gum guggul (2g 3x daily), "fraction A" of petroleum ether extract of guggulu (0.5g 2x daily) on serum lipids of 40 obese, 40 hypercholesterolemic and 40 hyperlipemic cases were observed. "Fraction A" brought a significant reduction in serum cholesterol and serum total lipids over a treatment period of 21 days and results compare (+) with clofibrate.

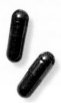

HERBAL PRODUCT TRIAL 1

❖ TITLE *Guggul as anti-inflammatory agent*

❖ SOURCE *Ind J Med Res (60(6), 926–39 1972*

❖ AUTHORS *Arora, R., Tanija, V., Sharma, Gupta*

❖ The steroidal fraction from the petroleum ether extract of the guggul showed significant effect on the primary as well as the secondary inflammation induced by Freund's adjuvant. It was more effective than hydrocortisone in reducing the severity of secondary lesions. Its antiphlogistic effect was comparable to that of hydrocortisone acetate.

HERBAL PRODUCT TRIAL 3

❖ TITLE *Study of Bringarja (eclipta alba) therapy on jaundice in children*

❖ SOURCE *J Sci Res plants Med 1981,2(4), 96–100 India*

❖ AUTHORS *Dixit, S., Achar, M.*

❖ In a trial 50 cases treated with E. alba powder (50 mg/kg body weight with honey) in 3 doses, 40 cases showed complete clinical and biochemical recovery from hepatitis in a period of 1–5 weeks. Pharmacological studies using alcoholic extract of plant showed antiviral activity.

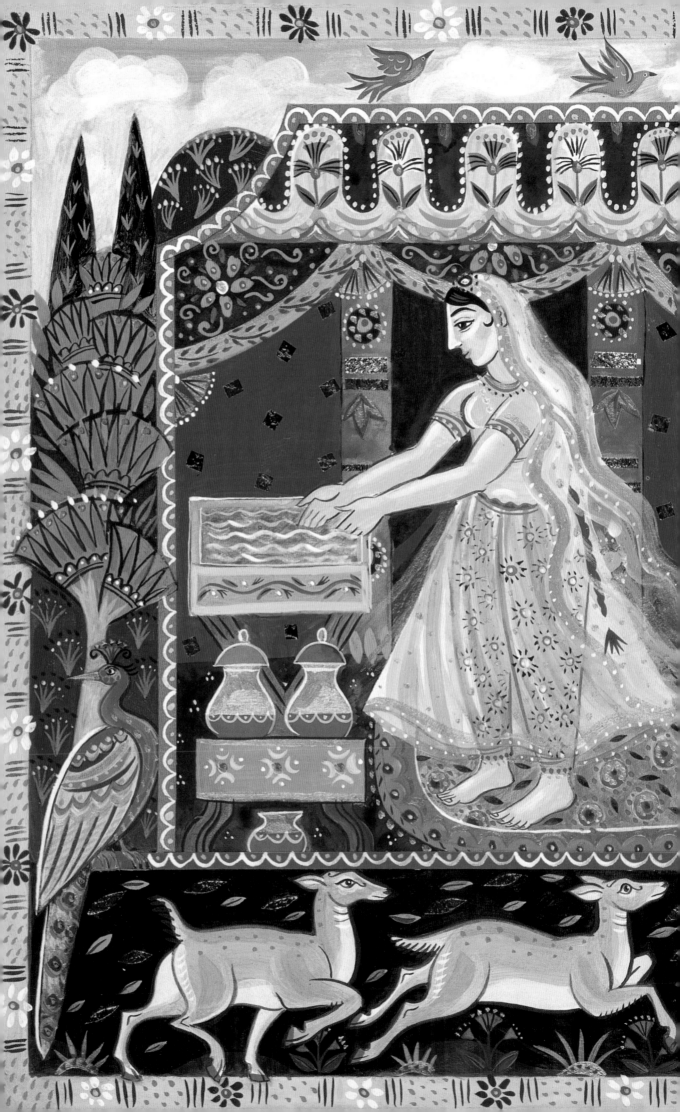

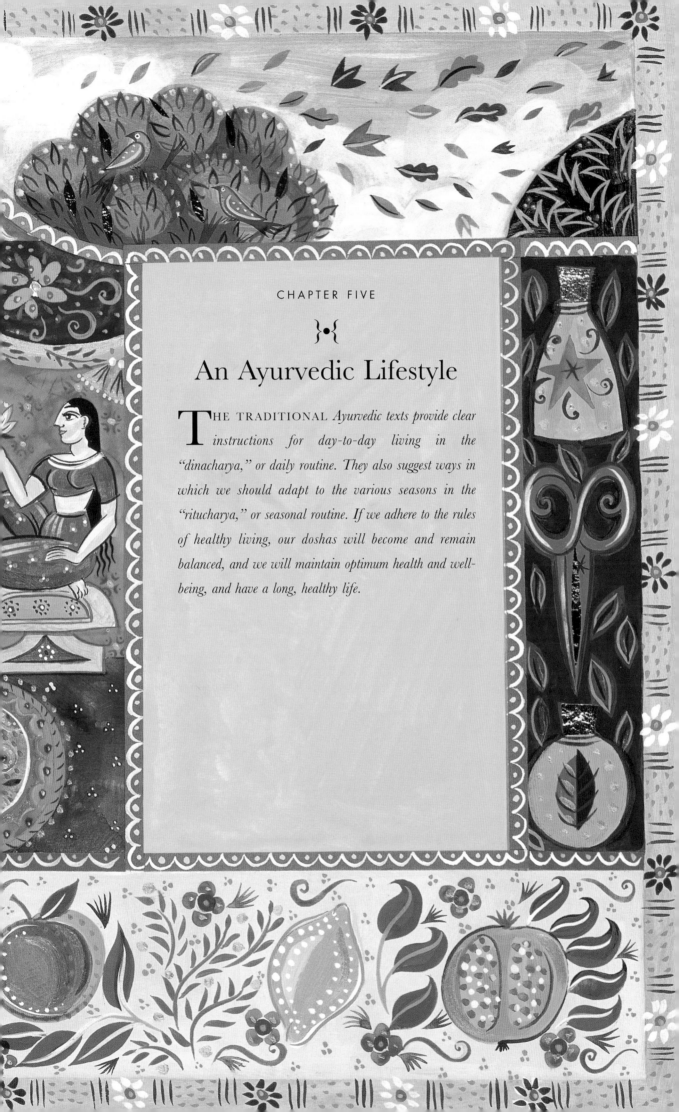

}•{

CHAPTER FIVE

An Ayurvedic Lifestyle

THE TRADITIONAL *Ayurvedic texts provide clear instructions for day-to-day living in the "dinacharya," or daily routine. They also suggest ways in which we should adapt to the various seasons in the "ritucharya," or seasonal routine. If we adhere to the rules of healthy living, our doshas will become and remain balanced, and we will maintain optimum health and well-being, and have a long, healthy life.*

Daily Routines ~ The Dinacharya

ALL THE AYURVEDIC classics give us detailed descriptions of how to maintain normal health through lifestyle. They tell us that "a wise man interested in long and healthy life, and who seeks happiness, must exercise the highest care in selecting what is wholesome in the matter of food, conduct, and behavior."

Charaka has given a comprehensive and detailed account of the mode of living and rules of good conduct to be followed if we want a good, healthy, and happy life. The average span of life for human beings should be one hundred years, but this may decrease if the prescribed good conduct is not adhered to.

Ayurveda believes that to achieve the fourfold objectives of life we must have good health. Those objectives are:

* Dharma (virtuous duty)
* Artha (wealth)
* Kama (enjoyment)
* Moksha (salvation)

In Ayurveda, hygiene, lifestyle, and diet are crucial to good health. To attain good health, Ayurveda prescribes the specific daily routine "dinacharya" and the seasonal regime "ritucharya." Before going any further, it is important to make clear what an Ayurvedic practitioner considers to be health.

Sushruta has defined health as "when the tridoshas are in a state of equilibrium, digestion, and metabolism is in order (agni), the tissue elements (dhatus) and excretions (malas) are in a normal state, and the individual is physically and mentally happy."

If you follow the prescribed regimen of life, and avoid the unwise course, you can be healthy and happy. Treatment is aimed at restoring the disturbed mechanism. The basic constitutional factors are the three doshas – vata, pitta, and kapha – and restoration of their dynamic balance regulates the life cycle and controls the entire body.

In Ayurveda, good digestion is the key to good health. Poor digestion produces "ama," a toxic substance believed to be the cause of illness. Ama is seen in the body as a white coating on the tongue, but it can also line the colon and clog blood vessels. Ama occurs when the metabolism is impaired due to an imbalance of agni.

Agni is the fire which, when working normally, maintains normality in all functions. Imbalanced agni is caused by imbalances in the doshas, and by such things as eating and drinking too much of the wrong foods and repressing emotions. Agni affected by too much kapha can slow the digestive process, making you feel heavy and sluggish, while too much vata can lead to wind, cramps, and alternate constipation and diarrhea. Agni also ensures that the three malas work effectively (*see* page 92).

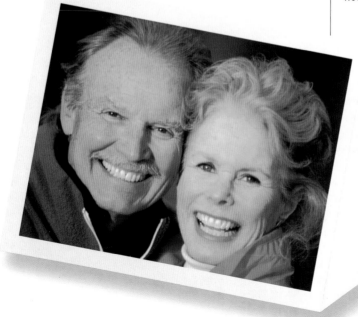

LEFT *Good diet, conduct, and behavior will help maintain health in later life.*

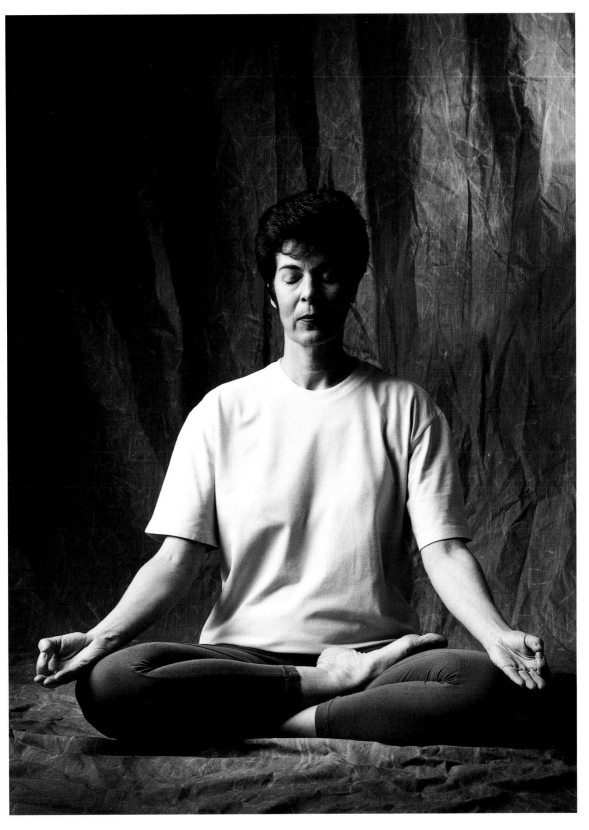

ABOVE *As part of the daily routine yoga and meditation help to maintain mental and physical balance.*

In the dinacharya or daily routine, it is most important that food is taken in a proper way, with regard to quality, quantity, and frequency. Ayurveda says that "food is the principal factor that materially contributes to the strength, complexion, and vitality of human beings." Diseases are believed to result from impaired nutrition. Food that is digested in due time without disturbing the equilibrium of doshas and dhatus (*see* page 93), and without impairing one's health, is regarded as the proper quantity of food. Ayurveda classifies food products according to their nature and qualities. Some foods are of vatika type (vata), so if a vatika individual consumes more vatika food, there is a possibility of increased vatika activity. Similar rules follow for the kaphaja (kapha) and paittika (pitta) types of food and individual.

Good health, according to Ayurvedic philosophy, is a state of balance between the mind, body, spirit, and environment. This balance, or harmony, is achieved through diet, exercise, lifestyle, meditation, the maintenance of psychological well-being, and the serenity that comes with self-acceptance.

Moreover, dietary rules need to be considered in relation to the seasons and times of the day. For example, a paittika diet should not be consumed in the summer or at midday when the paittika activity of the body is dominant.

THE THREE MALAS

Malas are the various waste products of the dhatus, produced during the normal metabolic processes. The three primary malas are purisha (feces), mutra (urine), and sweda (sweat).

It is clearly stated in the Ayurvedic texts that the balanced condition of the doshas, the dhatus, and the malas is good health or a condition free from diseases (arogya). Their imbalance is ill health or disease.

Purisha is the waste left when the nutrients of digested food have been absorbed in the small intestine. More water and salts are absorbed in the large intestine, and the residue, converted into solid feces, leaves the body.

The consistency of feces depends on the gastrointestinal mobility, and also on the nature of the diet. A vegetarian diet contributes to a larger bulk of softer feces, while a meat diet produces a smaller quantity of hard stool.

The tridoshas must be in balance to ensure normal evacuation. Pitta and kapha help digestion, and vata governs the mobility of the gut throughout the process. Any discrepancy or imbalance between these can lead to various symptoms of the gastrointestinal tract (e.g., a feeling of abdominal heaviness, pain in the abdomen, flatulence, constipation, and diarrhea), and may also give rise to such diseases as rheumatoid arthritis, osteoarthritis, low back pain, dysmenorrhea, asthma, bronchitis, as well as digestive problems such as stomach ulcers, irritable bowels, and constipation.

Mutra, or urine, is the mala derived during the course of biological processes taking place in the human body. The first stage of urine formation begins in the large intestine where fluids are absorbed into the system.

The entire urinary system (the kidneys, ureters, bladder, and urethra) takes part in the formation and elimination of urine, regulating the fluid balance in our body and also maintaining blood pressure. An imbalance, i.e., increased or decreased urine, results in various disorders, such as kidney stones, urinary infections, cystitis, abdominal pain, and bladder disorders.

Sweda (sweat or perspiration) is the third primary mala, and it occurs as a waste product during the synthesis of the meda dhuta (fatty tissue). Sweda, which is eliminated through the skin pores, controls body temperature, and helps to regulate electrolyte balance.

The channels that are responsible for bringing the sweat to the skin surface are known as sveda vaha srotas. It is essential that normal formation and flow of sweat takes place, as otherwise it can lead to a number of ailments like skin infections, dryness of skin, itching, burning sensation all over the body, loss of fluid balance, and reduced body temperature.

The dhatus support the mind as well as the body.

Rakta dhatu nourishes the body tissues and provides strength.

Asthi dhatu is the bone tissue, including the cartilage.

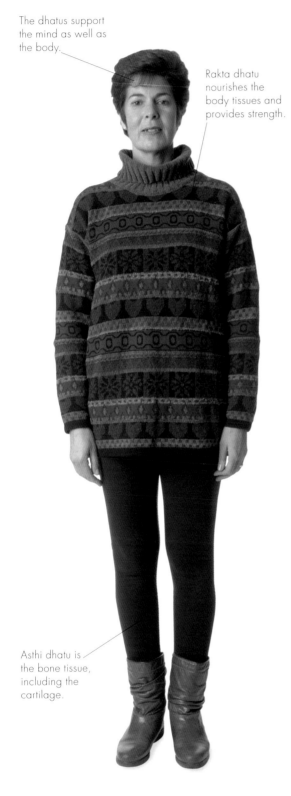

ABOVE *The sapta dhatus, or seven tissues, are known in Ayurveda as the pillars of the body, as they nourish and support.*

SAPTA DHATUS – THE SEVEN TISSUES

The seven tissue elements or dhatus, are the pillars of the body. Dhatu literally means to nourish or to support. The dhatus promote the growth of the body and support the body as well as the mind.

The seven dhatus are:

Rasa dhatu – This is derived from digested food, and nourishes each and every tissue and cell of the body. It is analogous to the plasma.

Rakta dhatu – Regarded as the basis for life, rakta dhatu is analogous to the circulating blood cells. It not only nourishes the body tissues but provides physical strength and color to the body.

Mamsa dhatu – This is the muscle tissue. Its main function is to provide physical strength and support for the meda dhatu (the adipose tissue).

Meda dhatu – The adipose tissue that provides support to the asthi dhatu (bone tissue). It also lubricates the body.

Asthi dhatu – Consists of the bone tissue, including the cartilage. Its main function is to give support and nourishment to the majja dhatu (bone marrow) and provide support to mamsa dhatu (muscle tissue).

Majja dhatu – The yellow and red bone marrow tissue. Its main function is to fill up the asthi (bone) and to oleate the body.

Sukra dhatu – The reproductive tissue. Its main aim is to help reproduction and strengthen the body.

Imbalance in the doshas also causes imbalance in the dhatus. The dhatus support and derive energy from each other, so when one is affected, the others also suffer. For example, interference in the manufacture of plasma affects the quality of the blood, which in turn affects the muscles. Each tissue type has its own agni, which determines the metabolic changes in the tissues. Each tissue also produces by-products, which are either used in the body or excreted. Menstrual periods, for example, are a by-product of rasa. The tissues are also governed by the three doshas so that heavy periods can be caused by the effects of excess kapha on plasma.

The daily routine as advocated in Ayurvedic classics can be summarized like this:

- **Early rising** An individual should get up early in the morning before sunrise (Brahma muhurta) and follow the regimen of:
- **Cleanliness** We have to take care of our bodies to keep them healthy. Clean habits are important, such as brushing the teeth; scraping the tongue; gargling and cleansing the mouth; regular massage of the body; application of oil on the head; bathing; trimming of beards, hair, and nails; ablution of the feet and the excretory orifices; wearing clean clothes; the use of scents, perfumes, ornaments, and footwear, etc.
- **Exercise** Properly performed exercise helps to keep you healthy and enables you to be happy both physically and mentally. To avoid harm, the type of physical exercise should depend upon your age and prakrti. Kaphaja persons should perform heavy exercise; paittika individuals should do it in moderation, avoiding exercise at midday and in hot seasons. Vata people should have regulated exercise in moderation, preferably yoga, and *not* aerobic exercise.

Exercise is not good for very weak and emaciated people, or after heavy meals, or for anyone who is in a febrile condition. It is strictly contraindicated for people who have bleeding tendencies, tuberculosis, heart diseases, asthma, or vertigo.

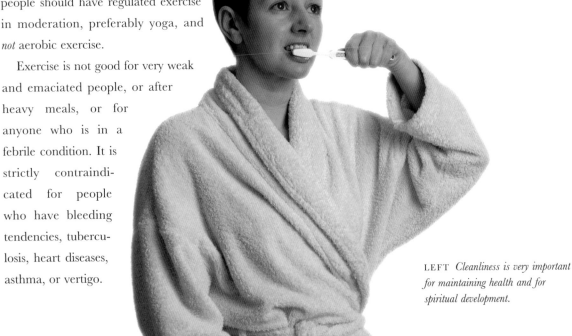

- **Satisfying natural urges** It is also important as part of your daily regimen not to suppress certain natural physical urges like urination, defecation, hunger, thirst, sleep, sneezing, eructation, yawning, vomiting, flatus, ejaculation, and panting. For good health you should satisfy these natural urges instantly, otherwise various diseases (related to the natural urge) may occur. For example, suppression of the urge for urination causes pain in the bladder and phallus, dysuria and distension of the lower abdomen. Suppression of the urge for defecation

LEFT *Cleanliness is very important for maintaining health and for spiritual development.*

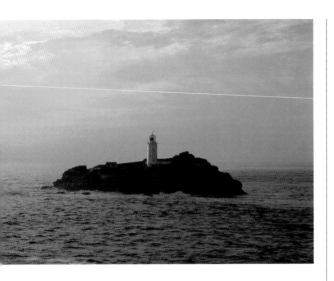

Strict mental discipline and strict adherence to moral values are considered vital to mental health. It is interesting that the key proponents of Ayurveda have long been aware that abnormal codes of conduct produce stress, and that errors of judgment are at the root of all stress. An improved code of conduct can free the body and mind from physical and mental disorders, preventing stress.

causes colic pain, headache, retention of feces, flatulence, cramps in the abdomen, and griping pain. Similarly, suppression of other urges leads to various complications or diseases. The daily regimen does recommend suppression of harmful psychic urges like greed, fear, anger, vanity, jealousy, malice, and excessive attachment to anything.

✣ **Mental and moral discipline** An equally important aspect of the daily regimen concerns mental health for which a regimen of sadvrtta is prescribed.

According to the daily routine, we should exert mental and moral discipline in the following ways:

✣ Respect God, teachers, saints, and elderly persons

✣ Be of help to others in times of difficulty

✣ Make firm decisions, be fearless, intelligent, brave, and of a forgiving nature

✣ Avoid fools, sinners, and people of a greedy nature

✣ Avoid undesirable places and excessive alcohol

EXERCISE

✤ **Charaka defined physical exercise as "that physical action or activity of the body that is desirable and capable of bringing about bodily stability and strength." It should be practiced regularly in the right measure.**

✤ **The good effects of taking exercise are lightness, capacity for work, firmness, tolerance of hardship, subsidence of humoral discordance, and stimulation of gastric fire or power of digestion.**

✤ **Too much exercise causes "fatigue, exhaustion, wasting, thirst, asthma, cough, fever, and vomiting."**

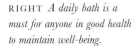

RIGHT *A daily bath is a must for anyone in good health to maintain well-being.*

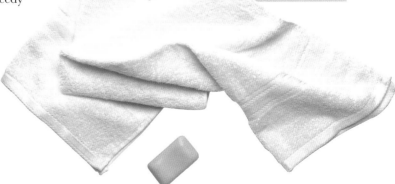

Seasonal Routines ~ The Ritucharya

AYURVEDA deals with the entire nature of life – good or bad, happy or unhappy, wholesome or unwholesome. A healthy person should follow the Ayurvedic seasonal regimen. Those who know the suitable diet and regimen for every season and practice these accordingly will experience enhanced strength and energy.

Before the seasonal ritual can be undertaken, it is important to understand the seasons themselves. The whole year is divided into six seasons: sisira rtu (late winter), vasanta rtu (spring), grisma rtu (summer), varsa rtu (rainy season), sarad rtu (fall), and hemanta rtu (early winter). The following table (from Charaka) shows the months according to the Hindu and the Western calendars.

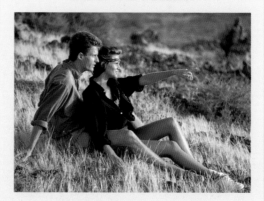

LIFE REGIMEN

For each season a detailed life regimen has been prescribed in all three Ayurvedic classics. Correct diet (anna), mode of living (vihara), and routine living (carya) will keep your doshas in a state of equilibrium (dosha samyawastha), helping you to cope with the stresses of the changing seasons.

ABOVE RIGHT *Understanding and enjoying the seasons for their different qualities is part of the seasonal routine of Ayurveda.*

HINDU AND WESTERN SEASONS

PERIOD	SEASONS	MONTHS ACCORDING TO HINDU CALENDAR	MONTHS ACCORDING TO WESTERN CALENDAR
Adana kala or period of dehydration	Sisira *late winter*	Magha and Phalguna	January – February February – March
	Vasanta *spring*	Caitra and Vaishaka	March – April April – May
	Grisma *summer*	Jyaishtha and Asadha	May – June June – July
Visarga kala or period of hydration	Varsa *rainy season*	Sravana and Bhadra	July – August August – September
	Sarad *fall*	Asvina and Kartika	September – October October – November
	Hemanta *early winter*	Magha and Pausa	November – December December – January

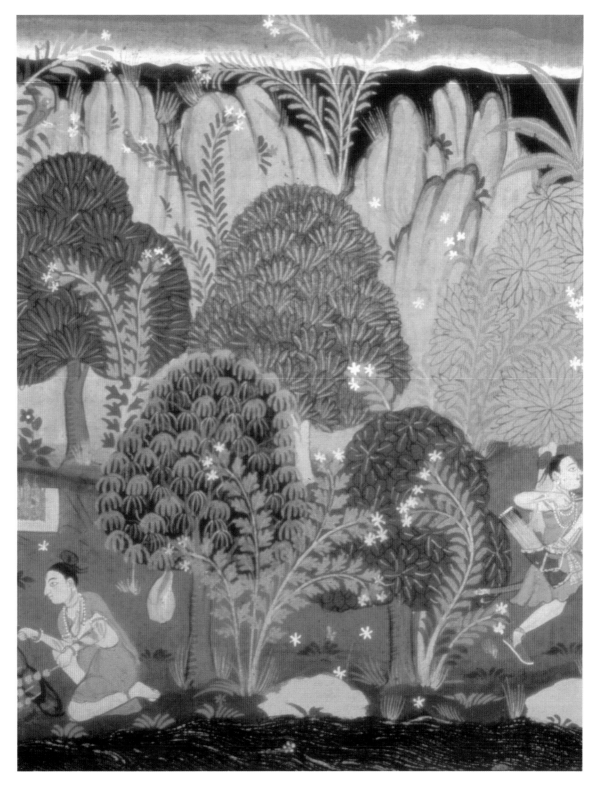

ABOVE *Appreciation of nature is the beginning of the understanding of Ayurveda.*

How the Seasons Affect the Tridoshas

The tridoshas are very much affected by the seasons. Vata is influenced more by early winter and the rainy season; pitta increases in summer, while kapha increases during the late winter. Therefore your diet and routine should take account of the seasons. A vatika diet should not be followed in the rainy season when the vatika activity of the body is already influenced by the season. Similarly, a paittika diet should not be consumed during summer, when paittika activity is at its peak. A kaphaja diet should be avoided in winter.

In the hydration period (visarga kala) winds are not as dry as in the period of dehydration (adana kala). During the period of dehydration not only the sun but also strong dry winds absorb moisture because of their sharp velocity and dryness, bringing about dryness in the atmosphere during late winter, spring, and summer. These drying effects cause physical weakness.

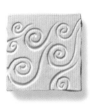

AIR

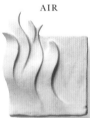

FIRE

WATER

DIETS

To provide generalized diets in the guise of precise dietary instructions for vata, pitta, and kapha in a book is not of much real value, as no one is ever of mono-doshic prakrti. It requires the assistance of an experienced Ayurvedic physician to assess the individual, as everyone's doshic equation is unique. This is why an old Ayurvedic proverb says "Ayurveda treats the patient, not the disease." The following dietary advice should serve only as a general guide for people with strong doshic personalities, before they have been assessed by a qualified practitioner.

PAITTIKA DIET

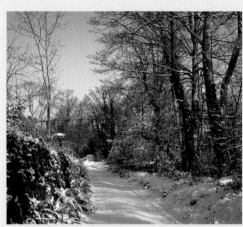

Recommended	Best Avoided
Milk	Yogurt
Butter	Sour cream
Apples	Lemons
Avocado	Bananas
Watermelon	Papaya
Sweet plums	Garlic
Lettuce	Leeks
Okra	Radishes
Cabbage	Almonds
Spinach	Cashew Nuts
Eggs	Most peppers and chilies
Fish	
Chicken	Very hot and spicy food
Garbanzo beans (Chick peas)	
Wheat	
Rice	
Oats	

During the period of hydration (which includes the rainy season, fall, and early winter), the rainwater helps to relieve the earth of the excessive heat, thus causing oiliness in the human body and stimulating growth and strength.

Late winter, the first season of the period of dehydration, is conducive to strength and good

VATIKA DIET

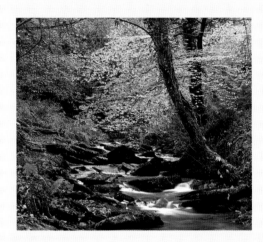

Recommended	Best Avoided
Milk	Yogurt
Buttermilk	Cabbage
Ghee	Cauliflower
Okra	Leeks
Green beans	Peas
Eggs	Potatoes
Fish	Spinach
Basmati rice	Pepper
Oats	Garbanzo beans (Chick peas)
Almonds	Kidney beans
Sunflower seeds	Turkey
	Cold drinks
	Coffee

KAPHAJA DIET

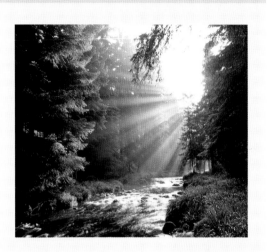

Recommended	Best Avoided
Apples	Milk
Apricots	Ghee
Peaches	Cheese
Broccoli	Avocado
Bitter gourd	Bananas
Cabbage	Dates
Garlic	Grapes
Chilies	Watermelon
Onions	Most sweeteners
Okra	Cold food
Most peppers and spices	Cashew nuts
Spinach	Peanuts
Tomatoes	Almonds
Chicken	
Fish	
Rice	

health. The second season (spring) gives rise to moderate strength and the third season (summer) causes weakness. This process is reversed during the hydration period so that the first season (rainy season) causes weakness, the second season (fall) gives moderate strength and the last season (early winter) is highly conducive to good health and strength. If you have gained enough strength during the last part of the period of hydration, you will continue to have some of it during the first season of the period of dehydration, but you will subsequently have lost your strength by the third season. Thereafter, the whole process is repeated, thus continuing the cycle.

An Ayurvedic Diet

DIET AND CONDUCT IN THE RAINY SEASON

The power of digestion is weakened during this period and the bodily vata is also aggravated. It is advisable to be moderate in your diet. Astringent, bitter, and pungent foods should be eaten. Water should be boiled, cooled, and mixed with a little honey.

In order to maintain normal powers of digestion you should take wheat and rice *(oryza sativum)* along with vegetable soup (preferably vegetables belonging to the three tastes mentioned earlier). You should abstain from daytime sleep, moving in the sun, excessive physical exercise, or excessive indulgence in sex. It is also advisable to massage the body by applying oils and to take regular baths during the rainy season.

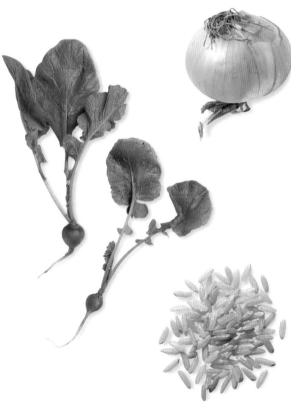

ABOVE *In order to maintain your health, it is very important that you vary your diet according to the season.*

DIET AND CONDUCT IN THE FALL

Food that is astringent, bitter, or sweet in taste, preparations of milk with sugar or honey, rice, barley, and wheat should be taken during this season. All kinds of water are recommended, as they are all clear and pure at this time of the year. In this season, sweet, light, cold, and bitter foods and drinks, which alleviate pitta, are to be taken in proper quantities. Ghee prepared with bitter medicines, purgation, and blood-letting are also recommended in the fall, to remedy the aggravated pitta of the previous season. Avoid excessive sunbathing, fat, oil, yogurt, and the meat of animals that live in water or marshy places. You should not sleep during the day, and should not expose yourself to frost or easterly winds. Exposure to autumnal flowers, sandalwood pastes, and to the rays of the moon in the evenings are all extremely beneficial. In short, all pitta-subduing measures should be resorted to in this season.

DIETARY CAUTION

All Ayurvedic diets prescribed for general use are ultimately of limited value because Ayurveda firmly believes that one person's meat is another's poison. Even two vata–pitta individuals may not thrive on the same diet because their vata/pitta/kapha equation may not be the same.

Therefore, all general diets should be approached with caution, particularly by those with any chronic or persistent complaints. The best way will be either to consult a qualified Ayurvedic physician, or to try a new food item (in very small quantities if you are ill) for a short while and to evaluate its effects before including it in your staple diet.

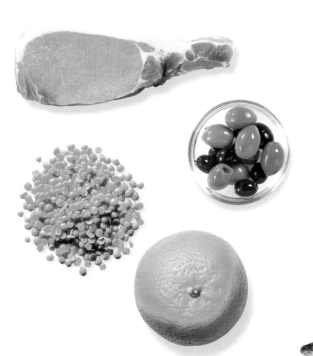

LEFT *Eat foods that avoid aggravating pitta in the fall.*

RIGHT AND BELOW *The meat of all aquatic animals should be avoided in fall, as should fruits such as pineapple.*

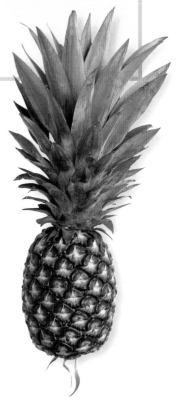

DIET AND CONDUCT IN THE WINTER

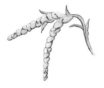

The winter season is cold but dry, the sun is weak, and the atmosphere cool and airy. Vata is aggravated during this season. Therefore during this season you should eat oily, sour, and salty food, and juices of the meat of aquatic and marshy animals. Food should not be taken cold. Preparations of cow's milk, cane juice, fat, oil, new rice, and hot water can improve your lifespan if taken regularly during the winter. Baths should be taken in tepid water after massaging your body with oils. Sufficient warm coverings for your body should be used. You can enjoy sexual pleasure intensely. You should avoid food and drink that are light and liable to vitiate vata, and so heavy food – both quantitatively and qualitatively – is prescribed for winter. You should not expose yourself to cold. This regimen holds good for both early winter and late winter (hemanta and sisira).

DIET AND CONDUCT IN THE SPRING

In spring, the kapha that has already accumulated is liquefied by the heat of the sun and, as such, disturbs your digestive capacity, causing many diseases. You should avoid eating heavy, oily, sour, and sweet food and drinks that may aggravate kapha. You should take food consisting of barley, wheat, and rice, and soup made of bitter vegetables. At the beginning of spring you should increase the amount of exercise that you do, have more massage with oils, and eat only light food. Those who cannot avoid smoking may smoke moderately at food time. You should not sleep during the daytime. Elimination therapies (panchakarma therapies, *see* page 154) consisting of emesis, purgation, decoction, oily enemas, and nasal errhines should be administered wisely. In short, it is wise to take measures that do not aggravate kapha.

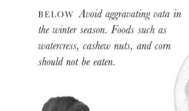

BELOW *Avoid aggravating vata in the winter season. Foods such as watercress, cashew nuts, and corn should not be eaten.*

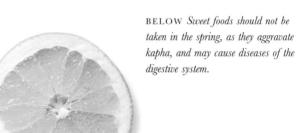

BELOW *Sweet foods should not be taken in the spring, as they aggravate kapha, and may cause diseases of the digestive system.*

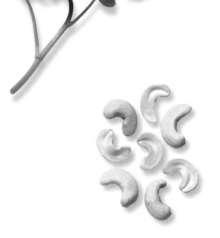

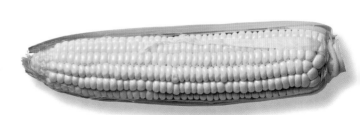

A DAILY ROUTINE IN THE SUMMER

The daily routine in the summer season follows very closely that of the winter season (*see* page 102), but with the following significant differences:

❖ Whereas some types of individuals can undertake heavy exercise in the winter, in the summer only mild physical exercise should be taken.

❖ No physical exercise is recommended for pitta prakrti individuals.

❖ Although you should not take an evening bath during winter, in summer a bath should be taken twice a day, and rather than tepid water, cold water should be used.

❖ It is important to drink plenty of fluids, including water, ghee, and milk.

❖ Eat the meat of animals or birds that inhabit areas with arid climates.

❖ Avoid foods, tastes, and regimens that aggravate pitta (*see* page 98).

❖ Try to take at least a short daytime rest.

DIET AND CONDUCT IN THE SUMMER

 During the summer, the strong sun evaporates the moisture of the earth, and so sweet, cold, liquid, and oily food and drinks are prescribed. You should avoid excessive physical exercise, hot and dehydrating food, and food with pungent, acid, and saline tastes. You should take plenty of water in general, and also with spirits if you drink alcohol as water helps to get rid of the alcohol's harmful effects. In India, those who regularly take cold mantha (a type of groat) along with sugar, as well as the meat of animals or birds of arid climate, ghee and milk along with sali rice *(oryza sativum)*, suffer no problems during the summer. During the daytime you should be in a cool environment. During the night it is recommended that you sleep in an open airy terrace of the house that is cooled naturally by the rays of the moon. You should avoid excessive sex and should enjoy the cool breezes of your garden, cold waters, and the fragrance of flowers of the season.

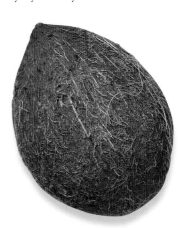

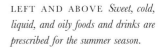

LEFT AND ABOVE *Sweet, cold, liquid, and oily foods and drinks are prescribed for the summer season.*

Disease Caused by Aggravated Vata

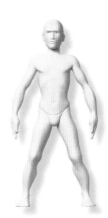

Vata is aggravated in the rainy season, fall, and early winter, and by all thought, eating habits, and behavior that increase vata in a person in whom vata is the dominant dosha.

An individual with vata as the dominant dosha will only suffer from vata-caused disease if the proportion of vata is out of balance with the other doshas. A significant increase of vata brought on by wrong food, extreme cold, or exposure to drafts can increase the incidence of disease.

Many people in Europe suffer from rheumatic and arthritic ailments because they attach too little importance to the cold and to over-exertion, which cause these vata-induced diseases.

CASE FILE

Sarah is a woman of 50, of medium height and somewhat overweight, who had been bedridden for over four months with a severe pain in her left thigh. This made it impossible for her to walk or to undertake any household work.

She works as a senior executive in a leading private-sector firm. After 20 years she was highly thought of in the company, which was very concerned about her health. A number of ultrasound and MRI scans, as well as consultations with rheumatologists and orthopedic surgeons, had not identified the problem, and Sarah had been on NSAID (Nonsteroidal and Anti-inflammatory) treatment for a number of months.

From her history, a visual examination, and a detailed examination of her stomach and limbs, it was clear that she was suffering from aggravated vata, and obstruction in the subtle nerve channels, causing severe pain in the left leg. She was also suffering from aggravated kapha, involving a hardening of the area.

This woman's history showed a consistent pattern of aggravation of her vata prakrti including:

❖ Eating vata-aggravating foods

❖ Keeping the house very cold, although she was sufficiently well-off to afford a warm house

❖ Exposure to drafts

❖ Emotionally upsetting relationship problems

Under such conditions any NSAID treatment would have aggravated her problem, and after four months of this treatment there was no improvement in her situation.

She was immediately prescribed:

❖ Massage with warm Chandanadi thailam (sandalwood-based oil)

❖ Guggul (*Commiphora mukul*) tablets

❖ Rasnadi kashayam (ingredients – *Alpinia galanga, Dasamoolam, Adhatoda vasica, Ricinus communis, Clerodendrum serratum, Homonoia riparia, Phyllanthas neiruri, Kaempferia galanga, Plumbago rosea, Cyperus rotundus, Phyllanthos emblica, Zingiber officinale, Oroxylum indicum, Trichosanthes cucumerina, Inula racamosa, Cedrus deodara, Chukrasia tabularis, Curcuma longa, Piper sp.*)

❖ Herbal sauna with Ashwagandha and Nirgundi herbs, and, after three weeks

❖ Vasti (enema)

Within one week her condition improved tremendously. Within three weeks she was walking. Now, after just six weeks of treatment, she is perfectly normal and back at work.

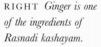

RIGHT *Ginger is one of the ingredients of Rasnadi kashayam.*

Emotionally upsetting relationships made her condition worse.

AGGRAVATED VATA

Rheumatism, rheumatoid arthritis, and all other musculoskeletal problems are caused by deranged vata, although the location of the ailment may be influenced by the other dominant dosha in the region. Deranged vata in the facial sinuses will cause kapha-related problems, including sinusitis.

❖ All musculoskeletal ailments and the inflammatory pain of rheumatic ailments are eased by applying heat, by vasti (herbal enema), and by massage with vata-reducing oils such as Narayana thailam and Sahacharadi thailam.

❖ Partial and full paralysis, and cardiovascular complaints in the elderly are all caused by excessively aggravated vata. The powerful force of aggravated vata, combined with ama (accumulated toxicity in the system) can unleash an upward movement of vayu, causing havoc in the central nervous and arterial systems. These are very serious ailments and need long-term (3–4 months) treatment with pizzchil (massage), vasti, and vata-reducing drugs like Guggul, Rasnadi kashayam, Maharasnadi kashayam, Narayana thailam, etc.

An examination of her stomach revealed aggravated vata.

❖ Aggravated vata can cause problems in the stomach and digestive system. These include obstructions in the stomach, severe pain, constipation, and the opposite, diarrhea.

Sarah had a severe pain in her left thigh.

❖ The best remedies for vata-related stomach and digestive problems are vata-reducing foods, aristhas such as Kutajarishtam and Mustarishtam, lehyas such as Vilwadi lehyam, and churnas like Hinguvachadi churnam.

Walking was difficult for Sarah until her Ayurvedic treatment.

RIGHT *Sarah responded very well to treatment. She is now walking normally and has returned to work.*

Disease Caused by Aggravated Pitta

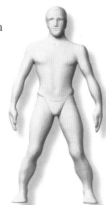

Pitta is aggravated in the late spring and in the summer and by thought, food, and behavior that increase pitta in a person for whom pitta predominates.

An individual with a pitta-dominant dosha may not suffer from pitta-caused disease as long as the proportion of pitta to the other doshas remains in balance. Increased intake of spicy food, lack of fresh air and cooling foods and activities, increased mental activity, and exposure to situations that provoke anger all aggravate pitta and can cause disease in a pitta-dominant person.

Two of the most common causes of increased pitta in Europe and the U.S.A. are over-exposure to the sun in the summer and drinking too little water.

CASE STUDY

This patient suffered from cystitis (muthra kricha), which is caused by increased pitta, complicated by vata.

Jane is a woman of 40 with one child. For ten years she had frequently suffered from cystitis that recurred every two to three months, causing her intense pain and suffering. She had passed blood through the urethra a number of times and each time had to be put onto Septrin, an antibiotic that is a mixture of sulphametuoxazole and trimethoprim. (By coincidence, a month after she stopped taking Septrin the drug was banned in the U.S. for causing leucopenia and severe allergic problems.)

Her history and examination revealed that a number of her habits were unfortunately conducive to causing cystitis including:

❖ Incorrect cleaning after defecation (pulling the toilet paper in the wrong direction)

❖ Using heavy douches to cleanse the vagina

❖ Baths with oils and soaps that irritated the urethra

❖ Lack of cleanliness after sex

❖ Insufficient consumption of water, particularly in summer

❖ Eating too much spicy food

She was asked to give up Septrin immediately and was prescribed:

❖ Chandanasavam (ingredients – *Vitis vinifera, Wood fordia floribunda, Ficus religiosa, Gmelina arborea, Monochoria vaginalis, Kaemferia galanga, Cyperus rotundus,*

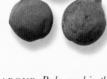

ABOVE *Beda, used in the treatment of aggravated pitta.*

Mangifera indica, Diospyros montana, Trichosanthes cucumerina, Oldenlandia corymbosa, Ficus benghalensis, Alpinia galanga, Santalim album, Glycyrrhiza glabra, Coleus zeylanicus, Bombax ceiba, Eugania jambolania, Andographis paniculata, Rubia cordifolia, Prunus puddum, Cyclea peltata, Pterocarpus santalinus)

❖ Chandraprabha vatika tablets (ingredients – *Acorus calamus, Andrograplus paniculata* (substitute – *Swetia chirata*), *Coscinium fennestratum* (substitute – *Berberis aristata*), *Aconitum farox* (now substituted because of non-availability), *Piper longum, Cyperus roaundus, Cedrus desdara, Curcuma longa, Piper nigrum, Baliospermum montanum, Ipomoes turpathum, Cinnamomum thanala, Elattaria cardamomum, Saccharum officinarum* (a source of sugar), *Comiphora mukul, Cinnamomum camphora)*

❖ Satavarigulam (ingredients – *Phyllanthus emblica, Groxylum indicum, Elettaria cardamomum, Santalum album, Glycyrrhiza glabra, Cynometra mimosoidas wall, Cinnamomum zeylanicum, Cuminum cyminum, Saussurea lappa, Coriandrum sativum, Cinnamomum tamala, Prunus puddum, Vattiveria zizanoiodes, Asperagus recamosus, Piper longum)*

❖ She was asked to drink at least 10 glasses of water a day and plenty of lime juice, and was advised to stop cleaning herself in the above-mentioned ways, including the use of the douche

❖ She was completely cleared of cystitis in two weeks

AGGRAVATED PITTA

All forms of hepatitis (A, B, Non-A, Non-B) are caused by aggravated pitta. The best Ayurvedic cure for hepatitis is medication containing *Cichorium intybus* and *Capparis spinosa*. Other treatments include virechan with Avipathi choornam, Parpatdyarishtam, and the Ayurvedic drug Liv 52.

❖ Excessive pitta causes skin problems, including psoriasis, burning sensation in the skin, skin eruptions, itching, and sores, which can become long term if complicated by kapha. The best treatment is the use of pitta-reducing kashayas (kwaths) such as Mahatiktaka kashyam, grithas such as Mahatikthaka gritham, and virechana with Avipathi choornam. Local application of Satowda gritham is very soothing and effective.

❖ Hyperacidity and gastric ulcers are a typical pitta problem, caused by increased secretion of stomach acid (pitta). A pitta type who is critical, ambitious, and irritable, and who abuses the stomach with spicy food, coffee, and tobacco will suffer from stomach ulcers. The treatment for ulcers and hyperacidity in Ayurveda is the intake of cooling and heavy products including buffalo milk, rice pudding, and ghee-based products like Mahatikthakam gritham.

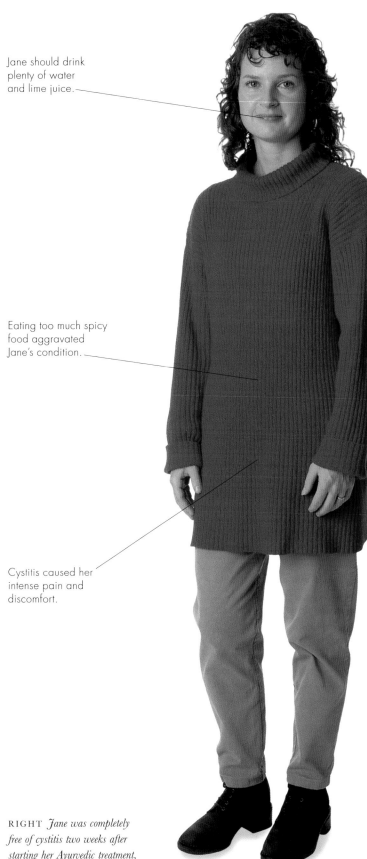

Jane should drink plenty of water and lime juice.

Eating too much spicy food aggravated Jane's condition.

Cystitis caused her intense pain and discomfort.

RIGHT *Jane was completely free of cystitis two weeks after starting her Ayurvedic treatment, and now has no pain.*

Disease Caused by Aggravated Kapha

Kapha is aggravated in the spring and in late winter, so foods and behavior that increase kapha should be avoided then.

An individual with predominant kapha will not suffer from kapha-caused illness if the proportion of kapha in relation to other doshas is in balance. However, a significant increase of kapha by overindulgence in sweet and oily food, excessive sleep or cold baths, lack of exercise, and exposure to cold will increase the incidence of disease caused by kapha.

Kapha-caused diseases tend to appear in infancy, pitta ailments increase at middle age, and vata-caused diseases often appear after middle age. Serious karmically inherited diseases (e.g., polio, blindness at birth) are exceptions to this rule. Asthma, eczema, and similar diseases attributed to allergy are caused by the kapha inherited from life in the womb.

CASE STUDY

The following case of childhood asthma illustrates the successful treatment of serious kapha-caused ailments through the use of Ayurvedic medicine.

Western medicine has traditionally believed that asthma is caused by allergy. Ayurvedic theory considers asthma to be entirely of kapha origin, a view that appears to have been confirmed by the medical establishment, which has only recently "unearthed" the implication of mucus in asthmatic disorders.

Katie is a young English girl of 12. She had suffered constantly from asthma for over eight years. Her medication had increased in strength from salbutamol tablets to Ventolin inhalers, steroid inhalers, and finally to frequent reliance on ventilators.

The girl was given vamana therapy, which brought out a considerable amount of mucus from the bronchial region. She was then given:

❖ Swasanandam gulika tablets (ingredients –
   Chayilam, Aconitum ferox, Cinnamomum,
   Terminalia chebula, Terminalia bellarica,
   Phyllanthes emblica)

❖ Chyavana prasam (ingredients –
   Dasamoolam, Sida rhambifolia,
   Cyperus rotandus, Cuminum
   cyminum, Microstylis wallichi,
   Kaempferia rotunda, Atylosia geonsis,
   Plantago amplexicaulis, Vitis cinifera, Elerraria
   cardomomum, Cinnamomum zeylanicum, Santalum
   album, Adhatoda vasica, Phyllanthes emblica,
   Ellettaria cardomomum, Cinnamomum tamala,
   Jaggery, ghee, oil, honey)

The course of treatment has brought about a dramatic improvement. She no longer has any need for the inhalers, but regularly takes Chyavana prasam, which has no long-term or short-term toxic effects and is also immunity enhancing.

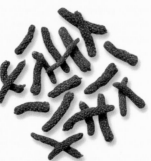

LEFT *Our patient has now stopped using her asthma inhaler.*

ABOVE *Jethimade is used to treat kapha-related diseases.*

LEFT *Diseases caused by aggravated kapha may be treated with Lindi pepper.*

AGGRAVATED KAPHA

Obesity is caused both by the kapha constitution and the individual's inherent attraction to food, particularly sweet and fried food. Serious obesity can cause major systemic problems including cardiovascular and musculoskeletal diseases. The right diet, regular yogic exercise, and Ayurvedic treatments such as massage, swedana (herbal sauna), and virechana combined with Guggul tablets will effectively reduce obesity and hypercholesaemia.

❖ Diabetes, one of the oldest diseases of mankind, is caused by excessive kapha. Lack of exercise, combined with over-indulgence in dairy products, meat, sweet-tasting food, and fried food, along with daytime sleep, increases kapha and can cause diabetes by middle age. Diabetes starts off as a kapha problem, exacerbates pitta and then vata to become a serious tridosha problem, difficult to cure. Early treatment by emesis and virechana therapy using Dhanwantaram ghee, and then regular intake of Khadiradi, Aragwadi, Kashayas, Chandraprapha gulika, Ayaskriti, Lohasava aristhas, Dhanwantaram, and Gulgulutikthaka grithams will eliminate diabetes in the early stages. Amrita choorna is also very effective for diabetes.

❖ Sinusitis is primarily a kapha problem, exacerbated by obstructed vata. The most effective treatment is Pratimarsha nasya with Anu thailam or Ksheerabala to penetrate the sinus cavity and bring out the sticky mucus. The patient should also receive kapha-reducing medications such as Thaleesapatradi vataka, Vasarishtam, Chyavana prasam, and Dasamoolarishtam.

Katie had suffered from asthma for over eight years.

Vamana therapy helped remove mucus from the bronchial region.

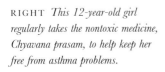

RIGHT *This 12-year-old girl regularly takes the nontoxic medicine, Chyavana prasam, to help keep her free from asthma problems.*

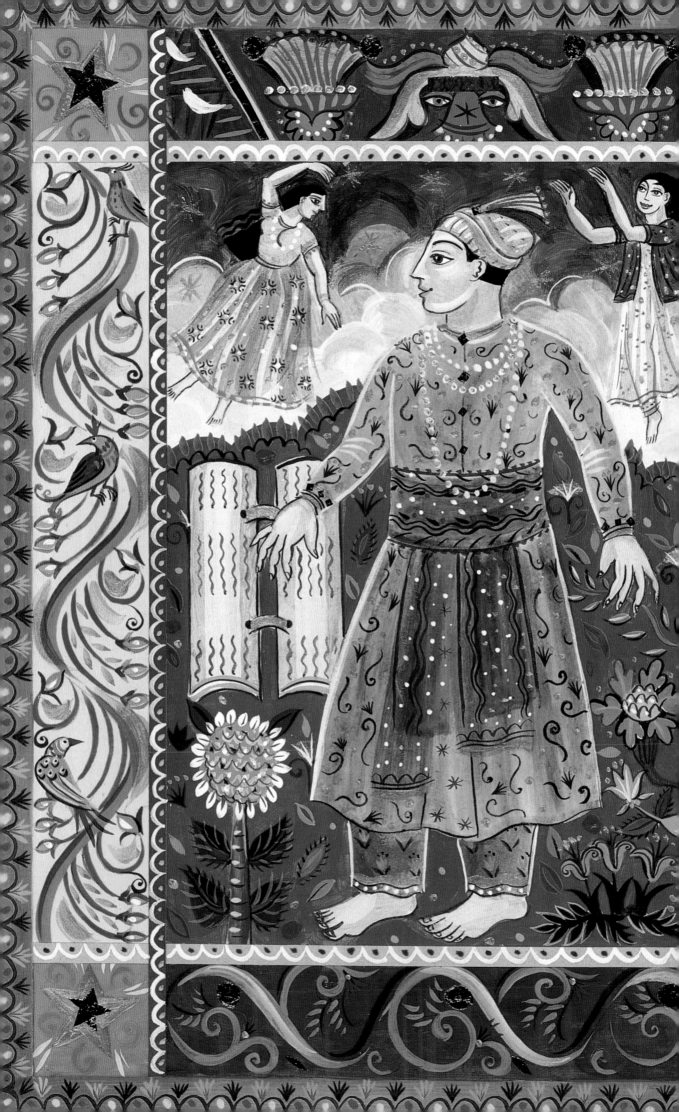

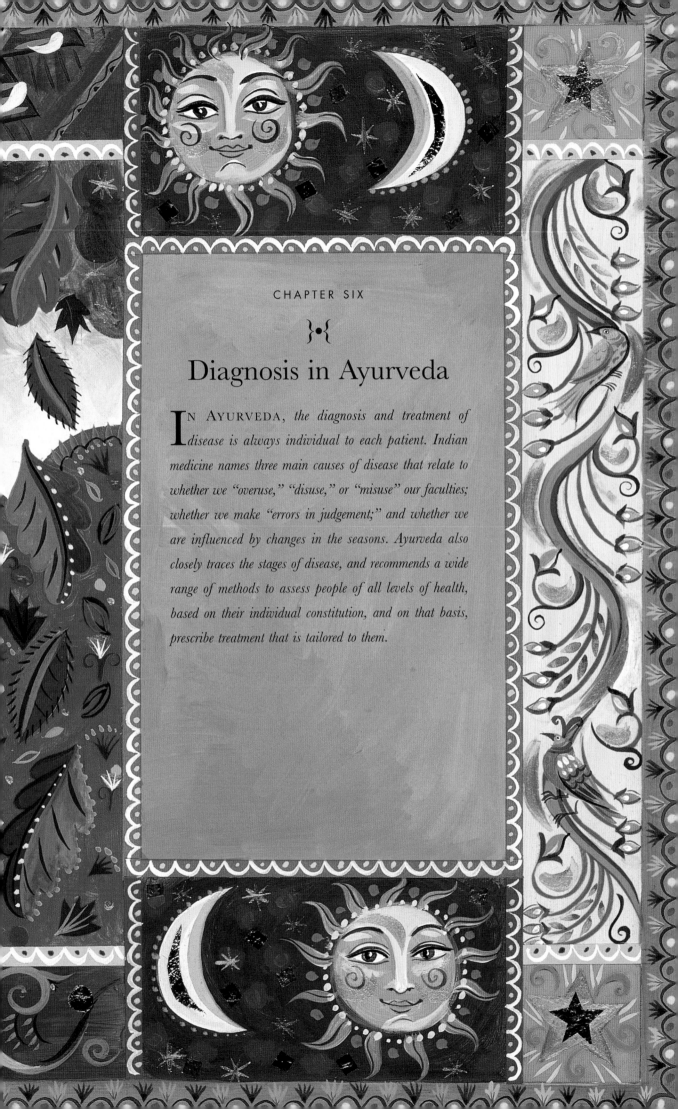

}·{

CHAPTER SIX

Diagnosis in Ayurveda

IN AYURVEDA, *the diagnosis and treatment of disease is always individual to each patient. Indian medicine names three main causes of disease that relate to whether we "overuse," "disuse," or "misuse" our faculties; whether we make "errors in judgement;" and whether we are influenced by changes in the seasons. Ayurveda also closely traces the stages of disease, and recommends a wide range of methods to assess people of all levels of health, based on their individual constitution, and on that basis, prescribe treatment that is tailored to them.*

The Three Causes of Disease

ACCORDING to Ayurveda an imbalance of the doshas that govern and indeed make up our physical and mental health is responsible for disease. Imbalance has three causes:

❀ The abnormal or unhealthy contact of sense organs with certain objects (asatmyendriyartha samyoga)

❀ Errors in judgement (prajnaparadha)

❀ The influence of time and the season (parinama)

Rightful perception is the result of coordinating your sensory apparatus with your

TASTE

mind and soul. As long as external stimuli are within normal limits, and the response of your body is also within physiological limits, it is suitable for your body and wholesome contact. But when stimuli exceed the normal range, they become stressful and the body's response is also an abnormal one. For example, if you subject yourself to long-term use of personal stereos at even normal levels of sound, this can seriously impair hearing over a period of time. This is excessive exposure to external stimuli.

TOUCH

SMELL

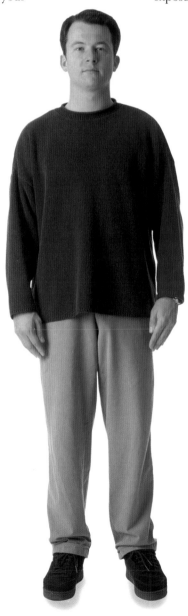

SIGHT

HEARING

GLOSSARY

Parinama

In common speech, parinama means "the result." Ayurveda believes that as a result of seasonal changes, specifically marked with traits that are contrary to its true nature, a number of diseases may arise.

LEFT *Rightful perception is the result of coordinating your sensory apparatus with your mind and soul.*

Stressful stimuli are the result of overuse, disuse, and misuse. For instance, with reference to light, it is considered "overuse" to gaze inordinately at excessively luminous objects; it is "disuse" to remain in complete darkness or not to look at anything at all; and it is "misuse" to gaze at objects that are either too close or too remote or frightful.

With reference to the sense of touch, it is overuse to expose yourself to extremes of climate and to indulge in excessive massage or baths; it is disuse to avoid all tactile stimuli; and it is misuse to resort to baths and to hot and cold applications outside the correct sequence (*see* pages 100–103) and to subject your tactile sense to contact with rough, uneven, and sharp surfaces or instruments.

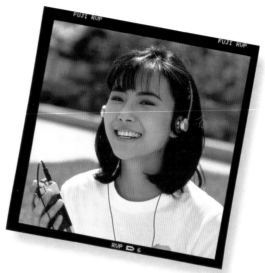

ABOVE *You should avoid exposing yourself to stressful stimuli, such as listening to loud music on personal stereos, for long periods.*

ASATMYENDRIYARTHA SAMYOGA

The five sensory organs of the human body – eye, ear, nose, tongue, and skin – help us with perception as they come in contact with the external world. Our sensory apparatus consists of:

✦ The five sense faculties, or pancindriya (which are visual, auditory, gustatory, olfactory, and tactual)
✦ The five sense organs, or pancindriya adhistana (which consist of the eyes, ears, nose, tastebuds or tongue, and the skin)
✦ The five sense substances or pancindriya dravyas (which consist of light, ether, earth, water, and air)
✦ The five sense objects or pancindriyarthas (which consist of shape, sound, smell, taste, and touch)
✦ The five sense perceptions or pancindriya buddhis (which consist of visual perception, auditory perception, olfactory perception, gustatory perception, and tactile perception)

PRAJNAPARADHA

This category includes all misconduct that follows from misconceptions of the intellect. Overuse, disuse, and misuse when it comes to body, mind, and speech lead to stress on the body and mind, ultimately causing imbalance of the doshas and development of disease.

For instance, misuse of your body includes suppression of natural urges, indulgence in rash acts, overindulgence in sex acts, moving in improper places and at improper times, and abusing the body. For example, if a man continuously restrains his urge to urinate, this will lead to bladder-related problems, such as cystitis, stones in the bladder, urinary infections, not to mention potential enlargement of the prostate.

Misuse of speech includes indulgence in language that is untrue, unpleasant, incoherent, harsh, untimely, or quarrelsome.

Misuse of your mind includes giving way to fear, grief, anger, greed, envy, infatuation, deluded thinking, or disrespect toward others.

In short, any act that is harmful to the body or any act arising out of passion and delusion is an error of judgment and causes disease.

PARINAMA

Seasons and other time factors are intimately related to the disease process, and we cannot ignore their impact on the human body. The year is broadly classified into three periods: winter, summer, and rain and snow.

When a season's characteristics are exaggerated, this is a "seasonal excess."

When its characteristics are less than normal, this is a "seasonal deficiency."

When a season has features that are contrary to its true nature, this is "seasonal abnormality."

So if a situation occurred where all these errors of seasons were present, it would result in an imbalance of the doshas and ultimately a manifestation of diseases as are common to the seasonal vagaries.

Besides these seasonal variations leading to imbalance of the doshas, it is interesting that there is another response of doshas to the seasons: day and night, intake of food, and age, so that some of the doshas become excited, some subdued. Under such circumstances, the diseases connected with those doshas can be triggered or made worse.

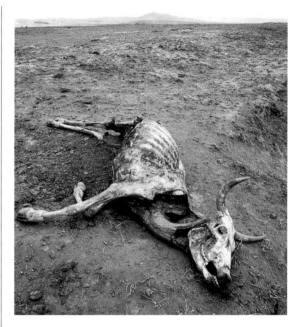

ABOVE *Periods of extreme weather conditions are termed "seasonal excess," and may have adverse effects on health.*

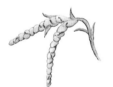   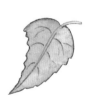 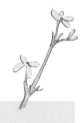

THE SEASONS AND THE DOSHAS

TIME FACTORS	EXCITATION OF VATA	EXCITATION OF PITTA	EXCITATION OF KAPHA
Season	Rainy	Fall	Spring
Day and Night (diurnal variation)	Afternoon Early night	Midday Midnight	Before noon Late night
Age	Old age	Adult age	Young age
Meals	After complete digestion of food	During the digestion of food	Just after taking meals

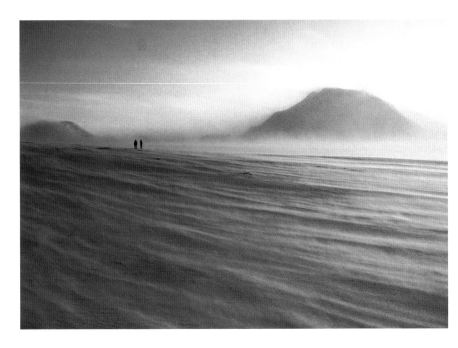

LEFT *The seasons are intimately related to disease and have a huge impact on the human body and its well-being.*

BELOW *In the early stages, correct treatment can prevent the doshas stagnating.*

THE RIGHT TIME FOR TREATMENT, OR KRIYAKALA

Imbalance of vata, pitta, and kapha is considered to be the immediate cause of all disease, and the factors that disturb them have already been discussed. A disease may subside after proper treatment or by natural efforts, but it may also remain in chronic form – or it may even prove fatal. Diseases proceed in distinct steps, and a good knowledge of the different (though modest) stages is necessary for the recognition of disease in its very early stages.

Kriyakala literally means "treatment period" or "time for action!"

Kala, or time, refers to the stages of disease, and the kriya, or action, signifies measures like medicine, diet, and lifestyle changes aimed at eliminating and correcting the doshic disturbances. If the doshas are checked or subdued in their first stage, the disease may not be able to proceed. But if left unremedied, they intensify and lead to the other stages. The six stages of kriyakala are:

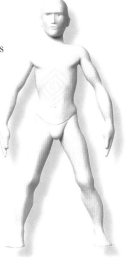

THE SIX STAGES	
Sanchaya	Stage 1
Prakopa	Stage 2
Prasara	Stage 3
Sthana samsraya	Stage 4
Vyakti	Stage 5
Bheda	Stage 6

The stage of sanchaya

This is the stage of accumulation of morbid doshas and is characterized by a vague and ill-defined set of symptoms. The doshas accumulate and stagnate in their own specific places and do not circulate freely. Symptoms characteristic of the dosha involved may sometimes be observed, for instance, a sense of dullness and fullness in the abdomen due to vata; yellowishness because of pitta; low body temperature and laziness or lethargy due to kapha. This stage involves aversion to similar things and attraction to contraries. Treatment should be started as soon as the specific symptoms appear, so as to avoid complications.

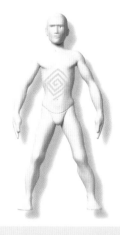

The stage of prakopa

In this stage the accumulated and stagnant doshas become "excited." The table below shows the exciting factors for each dosha, with reference to ahara, vihara, and seasonal and climatic states.

Diseases may become excited due to seasonal changes or wrong behavior. For example, a person who already suffers from mild stomach discomfort may overindulge in the wrong food and can have an acute episode.

SANCHAYA, PRAKOPA, AND PRASHAMA OF THREE DOSHAS IN VARIOUS SEASONS

	LATE WINTER	SPRING	SUMMER	RAINY SEASON	FALL	EARLY WINTER
Vata			Sanchaya	Prakopa	Prashama	
Pitta				Sanchaya	Prakopa	Prashama
Kapha	Sanchaya	Prakopa	Prashama			

Note: *Prashama means remission of the dosha if treatment or remedial measures are adopted. Otherwise the disease goes onto the prasara, or spreading, stage.*

AGGRAVATION OF DOSHAS BY FOOD AND ACTIVITY

DOSHA	FOOD	ACTIVITY
Vata	Intake of food having similar properties to vata – e.g. food and drinks having bitter, astringent, and pungent taste are known to excite vata. Ingestion of food substances such as dried leafy vegetables, such as lentils or beans, spinach, etc. Irregular eating habits, starvation and unbalanced diets.	Strenuous exercise, excessive running, swimming, keeping late hours, sexual excess, carrying heavy loads, suppression of natural urges – micturition, defecation, sneezing, etc.
Pitta	Intake of food having properties similar to pitta, e.g., food and drinks having sour, salty, and pungent taste. Among the articles of food that are known to excite pitta are sesame oil, mustard oil, curd, pepper, chilies, alcohol, fermented foodstuffs, some green leafy vegetables, and fruit such as amla.	Anger, grief, fear, unnatural modes of sexual indulgence, excessive exposure to the sun.
Kapha	Intake of such articles of foods that are possessed of heavy, cool, soft, greasy, sweet, and unctuous properties. Foods and drinks of sweet, sour, or salty taste cause excitation of kapha. Food substances such as butter, curd, milk, chocolates, sugar, and meat.	Day sleep, lazy and sedentary habits, repeated eating before the completion of digestion of previous food, etc. cause enormous accumulation or excitation of kapha.

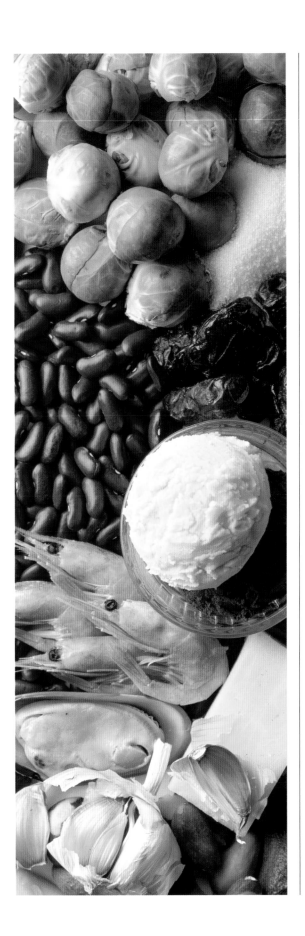

AGE

❖ Observance of right behavior in the seasons is the key to maintaining good health and curing disease. This applies not only to individuals with mild or serious ailments but particularly to the healthy. Most people have good health during their youth and in the early thirties, but it is in middle age that the signs of the body's misuse begin to manifest. This is because the early part of life is governed by kapha for all people and this kapha period provides general good health (apart from colds, skin problems, etc.) other than for a few unfortunate individuals. The middle part of life, which is governed by pitta, generally tends to manifest pitta-related ailments, such as stomach and digestive problems, ulcers etc. From the middle age onward, the wrong habits and misuse of early life begin to take their toll. Vata sets in and the unavoidable ailments of old age begin to take effect.

❖ The observance of ritucharya, the correct seasonal behavior unique to your own prakrti, helps to minimize a number of complaints caused by misuse, and even the severity of the natural problems of old age, such as rheumatism and arthritis. Correct living, combined with the practice of yoga and meditation, helps lead you gently and gracefully into vanaprastha, the period of spiritual retreat. In India it was traditional to leave your active life after a certain age (around 55 years old) to seek a more spiritual way of living. Fear of becoming old is always caused by attachment to material desires and by fear of illness and poverty. All these fears disappear into the mist as you gain peace and light through self-knowledge and through health derived from correct living. In other words, you must invest in your future, not by pensions, but by understanding your body and your true nature, which is none other than the cosmos itself.

The stage of prasara

The term "prasara" means to spread. At this stage the excited and accumulated doshas spread to other parts, organs, and systems of the body, leaving their original sites. This spread may be of a single dosha, or a combination of two or three may be simultaneously involved. The excited and aggravated doshas travel through the body, become confined to a particular part of the body, and may give rise to disease there.

Generally, up to the stage of sanchaya and prakopa, the damage is fully reversible and, with proper measures, the restoration of doshic balance may be achieved. Because the doshas are influenced by time and season, there may be spontaneous prashama (remission) at times. For instance, there is sanchaya of pitta in the rainy season, prakopa in fall, and prasara in early winter, etc. Depending upon the degree of excitation, it may pass to the stage of prashama (remission) or prasara (spread).

Sthana samsraya

This is the early phase of disease when the wandering doshas become localized in a particular tissue, organ, or system, giving rise to disease of those structures. For instance doshas, when confined to the abdomen, may give rise to constipation, diarrhea, impairment of digestion, abdominal tumors, and diseases of the liver, spleen, and other abdominal organs. Doshas, when confined to the urinary system, may give rise to urinary tract infections, retention of urine, renal calculi, and diabetes mellitus (meha).

The stage of vyakti

At this stage, the symptoms of fully developed disease are present. These include for example edema (sopha), pyrexia (jvara), or diarrhea (atisara).

The stage of bheda

In this stage the disease may become chronic or incurable. There are several diseases that are automatically taken care of by the body's defence mechanism and resistance, but if the body is incapable of fighting the disease, several complications may be produced. The necessity of recognizing this stage lies not only in its being a valuable aid for prognosis, but also in the fact that when the diseases come to this stage, they may act as predisposing factors for the spread of other diseases.

The careful analysis of the stages of kriyakala helps us to understand the phenomenon of disease, to make an early diagnosis, and to adopt preventive and curative measures to help the patient.

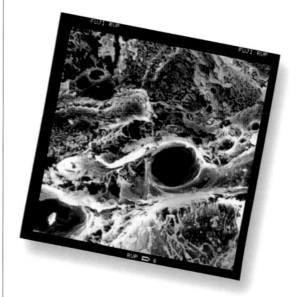

ABOVE LEFT *At the prasara stage, the aggravated and excited doshas leave their original site and spread to other parts of the body.*

ABOVE *A patient's disease may become chronic or incurable at the bheda stage, as in this case of advanced liver cirrhosis.*

This patient often suppressed his urge to urinate, causing cystitis and prostate problems.

The kidneys have become infected.

The patient has an enlarged prostate causing urinary retention.

RIGHT *If left untreated, a disease will spread and become more difficult to cure, as in this case of prostate enlargement.*

CASE STUDY

This case study illustrates how a particular disease develops (in this case prostate enlargement). Alan, a man in his 50s, who drove a lot for his living, began suffering from cystitis due to suppressing his urge to urinate. He sometimes took antibiotics, but often left the problem untreated. He did not refrain from sexual intercourse at this time, and due to his illness, often indulged in foreplay, without ejaculation. This resulted in prostatic fluid accumulating in the prostate. This is the sanchaya, or accumulation stage.

❖ His prostate became enlarged over a period of time. Eventually it reached a point where it began to obstruct urine flow, and his bladder expanded to accommodate more urine. Stones might now form in the urinary tract and the kidney itself become infected. He also experienced constipation due to the enlargement of the posterior part of the prostate. Now the total excretory system was affected leading to tridosha kopam, the aggravation of all three doshas. This is the prasara, or spread stage.

❖ By the bheda stage, the disease has become chronic and may be incurable. The prostate is heavily enlarged and urinary retention has intervened. Western physicians would normally catheterize the patient at this point to allow urine flow. This may in itself introduce infection into the urethra and the urinary tract. The urologist would now examine the patient with a cystoscope and possibly take an IVU (intravenous urography) to give a clear picture of the kidneys and the urinary tract. Transurethral resection of the prostate (TURP) would now be considered as there are no other treatments in Western medicine to reduce an enlarged prostate.

❖ However, even at this late stage, Ayurvedic treatment can help. A combination of Chandraprabha, Shatavarigulam, Chandanasavan, and Moothra vasti (introduction of Ayurvedic medicines through the urethra and the bladder into the prostate region) can still reduce the size of the prostate and clear the bladder and urinary tract of built-up doshic toxins.

Constitutional Treatment

CONSTITUTIONAL treatment in Ayurveda involves the careful examination of the patient according to the principles of Ayurveda. A diagnosis of the precise nature of the doshic imbalance can be made by taking the patient's history, performing the eightfold examination, and assessing the patient's specific symptoms. The good Ayurvedic physician will also

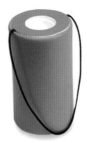

ABOVE *The patient's lifestyle and work must be taken into consideration.*

take into account the karmic and spiritual elements of the patient's disease, including the patient's astrological chart. He will then inquire about spiritual and religious practices, as well as the patient's general lifestyle. The primary objective of the constitutional treatment will be to rebalance the patient's doshas and not just to provide symptomatic relief.

CASE STUDY

Caroline is a 50-year-old charity worker. She complained of joint pain, especially in the knees and ankles. The pain was aggravated by excessive exercise, active movements, standing for long hours at charity balls, and exposure to cold. This pain initially started with the knee joint and gradually spread to other joints. Now very painful, there is a lot of redness and swelling in her joints. She also suffers from indigestion and variable appetite, as well as anxious and disturbed sleeping patterns.

Caroline has no other ailments and would lead a normal life if she did not have these joint pains. She is a vegetarian and normally has a balanced diet, though occasionally it becomes irregular due to her busy schedule. She is now gaining weight because of her restricted movement, and lack of exercise. Her grandmother and mother both had painful joints.

The eightfold physical examination revealed:

❖ Prakrti – vata kaphaja

❖ Sattva (mind) – normal, though stressed at times

❖ Bala (strength) – moderate

❖ Nadi (pulse) – vataja nadi (predominance of vata)

❖ Jivha (tongue) – dry, and coated at times

❖ Tvak (skin) – dry and rough

❖ Sabda (voice) – normal

❖ Drka (vision) – normal

❖ Akrti (appearance) – normal except for knee joints, which are slightly swollen

❖ Mala (stools)– irregular bowel habit

❖ Mutra (urine)– normal

Examination revealed swollen knee joints, other joints were not swollen.

Diagnosis – a case of Amavata

The following lifestyle recommendations were made:

❖ Adequate rest

❖ Regularizing her sleeping habits

❖ Avoidance of standing for long hours

❖ Meditation to control anxiety

❖ Diet

❖ Vata-pacifying diet (*see* page 164)

❖ Avoidance of irregular meals and fasting

❖ Easily digestible food

She was also treated with guggul and ama pachak medicine to promote and correct digestion, and prevent the production of ama, the factor responsible for this particular disease.

Once the swelling subsided, Caroline was treated with panchakarma treatments. Snehana, swedana, virechana, and vasti therapies were given at appropriate intervals and with the proper pre- and post-panchakarma measures. She was also massaged with Mahanarayana taila oil.

Caroline responded extremely well to her drug, dietary, panchakarma, and lifestyle recommendations, and there has been no recurrence of her joint pain since.

Meditation helped Caroline to control her anxiety.

A vata-pacifying diet was recommended as part of the treatment.

Caroline's pain started in the knees but soon spread to other joints.

Standing for long periods aggravates joint pain.

RIGHT *A combination of Ayurvedic drugs and lifestyle recommendations helped rid Caroline of her joint pain.*

THE THREE DOSHAS AND THEIR COMPOSITION

❖ Vata is a combination of air and space, and corresponds to the Anja chakra in the center of the forehead. Vata people are highly mobile, idealistic, creative, and tend to be escapist in attitude. Most artists and dancers have a high vata element. Unfortunately, very high vata, combined with pitta, can result in psychiatric illnesses. Most cases of mental ailment occur due to the inability of high vata individuals to integrate their basically escapist nature into the renunciation mode of spirituality necessary to balance the doshas and their minds. The best example is Lord Shiva himself. As Nataraja, he is the Lord of Dance, and all Indian dancers worship him before performing. His cosmic dance represents the dissolution of the universe, indicating the power of dynamic vata to destroy all existing structures, both physical and mental.

❖ Kapha is a combination of earth and water, and represents the Muladhara chakra in the kundalini. This chakra is also called the Brahma Granthi and represents the creator god Brahma. Located around the sexual and procreative organs, it is directed toward creative activity, making kapha people the most solid and earthy of the three dosha types. A high amount of kapha is necessary for material success in the world. Kapha–pitta types successfully balance material and spiritual orientations, making them both responsible and compassionate.

❖ Pitta is the combination of fire and water, and represents the Manipura chakra in the kundalini, located around the navel. It represents Lord Vishnu, the preserver, who balances the forces of Creation, i.e., the kapha and the vata tendencies. Pitta individuals have a very high drive, a fanatical commitment to causes, and are aggressive and ambitious. Lord Vishnu himself is more pitta–kapha in nature, balancing the intellectual aspects of pitta with the loving aspect of kapha. Most cult leaders and ambitious businessmen and women will have high pitta doshas. However, if they have vata as a secondary dosha, they tend to become careless of ethics and social responsibilities.

Diagnostic Techniques

EXAMINATION OF THE PATIENT

Ayurveda believes that the imbalance of vata, pitta, and kapha doshas causes disease. As long as these three remain in complete harmony, the body is normal, but as soon as they become imbalanced (whether singly or in combination), disease follows. The examination of the patient consists of the following methods of diagnosis:

Causes of disease, or nidana

It is important to assess the causes of disease in order to understand the illness, to select remedial measures, and, of course, to prevent recurrence. If the causes remain after therapy has been initiated, the response will be quite unsatisfactory and recurrence will take place. On the other hand, if the causes are understood properly, it is possible to remove them, assisting recovery.

Early signs and symptoms, or purvaroopa

The early symptoms give us useful warnings and signals before a disease is fully manifested, so that we can work to avert it or at least to reduce the symptoms of that illness.

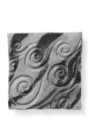 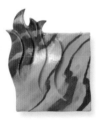 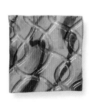

AIR   FIRE   WATER

Main signs and symptoms, or roopa

The signs and symptoms of the fully developed disease reveal which doshas are involved, as well as the intensity and prognosis of the disease.

Exploratory therapy, or upasaya

This includes measures such as medicine, diet, and routines to help identify diseases that are otherwise difficult to diagnose. These measures either act directly against the cause of the disease, or the disease itself, or they produce relief. For instance, if a swelling is alleviated by a massage with oily and hot things, the swelling is caused by imbalance of vata (*see* page 56).

The production of disease, or samprapti

The imbalance of the doshas and the course that they follow to cause disease is termed as samprapti, or pathogenesis.

ENTERING THE MIND

Charaka emphasized in his text that if a physician is not able to enter into the mind of his patients, he cannot treat them with positive results.

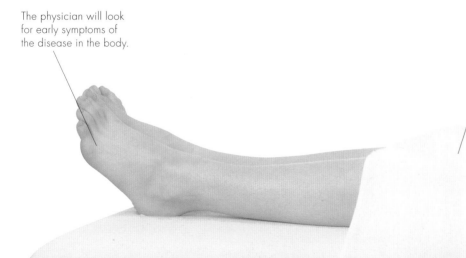

The physician will look for early symptoms of the disease in the body.

Imbalance of vata, pitta, and kapha doshas causes disease.

CLINICAL EXAMINATION OF THE PATIENT

Clinical examination of the patient is important for correct diagnosis and treatment of disease. Many people are reluctant to reveal fully their symptoms and personal problems, so the physician has to gain the patient's confidence through suitable conversation and appropriate clinical examination in order to treat the patient successfully (*see* page 120, Constitutional Treatment).

Textual knowledge (aptopadesa), direct perception (pratyaksha), and inference (anumana) are all important to clinical examination. These three should be methodically and meticulously used in order to examine the patient and to arrive at the correct diagnosis.

Textual knowledge and our understanding of medicinal preparations help us to interpret diseases that have been studied in detail for centuries – for example, their exciting causes, involved doshas, complaints, symptoms, physical signs, prognosis, and diagnosis.

Knowledge obtained through the patient's own perceptions and experience also helps the physician. This includes the patient listening to their body, inspection, and palpation.

Inference usually involves assessing the strength of the patient (by his or her capacity to perform exercise or work); digestive fire (by the patient's power of digestion); clarity of sense organs (by the power of perception); mind (by the power of concentration); the capacity of understanding (by purposeful action); anger (from actions of violence); and pleasure (from the sense of satisfaction).

Examination of patients may involve the tenfold examination (dashvidha pariksha, *see* page 124) and/or the eightfold examination (astavidha pariksha, *see* page 128). These help to evaluate the strength of the patient and of the disease.

ABOVE AND LEFT *The clinical examination includes an assessment of the individual's personality and lifestyle.*

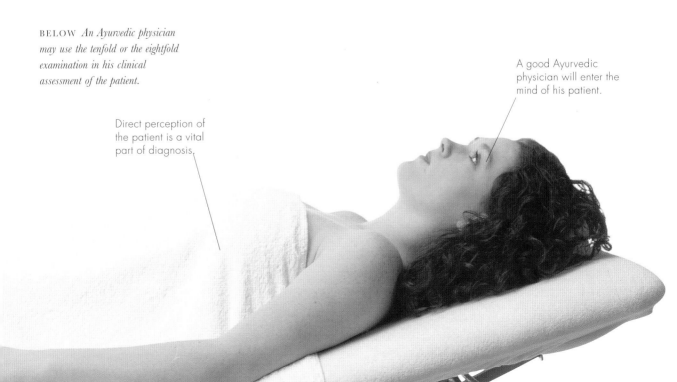

BELOW *An Ayurvedic physician may use the tenfold or the eightfold examination in his clinical assessment of the patient.*

A good Ayurvedic physician will enter the mind of his patient.

Direct perception of the patient is a vital part of diagnosis.

The Tenfold Examination

The tenfold examination, dashvidha pariksha, involves the following aspects:

❋ **Body constitution** (prakrti)
The body constitution is determined by genetic factors in the womb. The relative predominance of doshas during fetal development determines the prakrti (constitution), which may be vatika, paittika, kaphaja, vata paittika, vata kaphaja, pitta kaphaja, or samdoshaja (*see* page 67).

❋ **Pathological state** (vikrti)
In order to assess the strength of the disease, the causes, the doshas, the affected body elements, prakrti, time, and strength of an individual, the signs and symptoms of the disease have to be considered. This enables us to understand the disease in its entirety. The pathological state is related to the history of the patient and the physician's expertise and knowledge.

❋ **Tissue vitality** (sara)
Broadly speaking there are seven vital tissues: rasa (lymph), rakta (blood), mamsa (muscle), meda (adipose tissue), asthi (bone), majja (bone marrow), and sukra (reproductive tissue) (*see* page 93). The features of these tissue elements are examined in their respective sites.

The physician examines the features of rasa in the skin (tvak) by assessing its smoothness, softness, clearness, thinness, and whether it is covered with short, deep-rooted, and delicate hairs. A healthy skin will appear full of luster.

The evaluation of rakta (blood) depends on the condition of the eyes, mouth, tongue, lips, nails, hands, and the soles of the feet.

> ### YOUR CONSTITUTION
> **Though a healthy body requires equilibrium of the three doshas, there is always some variation of doshas in the body. Your prakrti is important for determining your susceptibility to different diseases, the general course the disease would adopt, the pattern of its presentation, complications, and the overall prognosis. Ultimately, all the measures of preservation of health and well-being, and the treatment of disease are based on consideration of your constitution.**

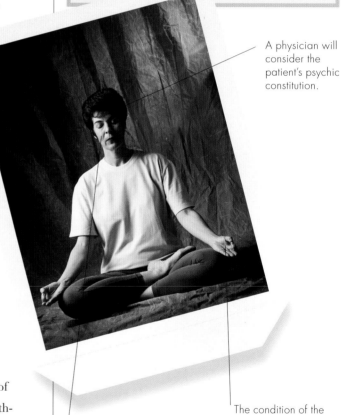

A physician will consider the patient's psychic constitution.

The condition of the hands is used to evaluate rakta (blood).

The physician will examine the skin for features of rasa (lymph).

ABOVE *A healthy mind and body are signs that the three doshas are in complete harmony.*

When the mamsa, or the muscular tissue is in perfect condition, the temples, forehead, nape of the neck, shoulders, belly, arms, chest, joints of the body, jaw, and cheeks are covered with firm and heavy muscular tissue.

People with healthy meda or adipose tissue have sufficient oiliness in their complexion, eyes, hair, nails, and lips, as well as a healthy voice and healthy teeth.

The health of asthi, or bony tissue, is shown by pliable but firm forearms, chin, nails, teeth, ankles, knees, and other joints of the body.

Those in whom the majja, or bone marrow, is in good health are strong and of good complexion and have stout, long, round, and stable joints.

Those in whom the sukra, or semen, is in perfect health are strong and cheerful. They have round, firm, close, and even teeth, good voice and complexion.

❀ **Physical build** (samhanana)
Body examination is done by direct perception. The healthy body is well-built, the bones are symmetrical, the joints are stable and strong with enough flesh and blood.

❀ **Body measurement** (pramana)
In Ayurveda, the body measurement is given in terms of finger breadth. A person having close proximity to these measurements is termed as normal and healthy.

BELOW *An experienced Ayurvedic physician will learn much about the patient's state of health from the tenfold examination.*

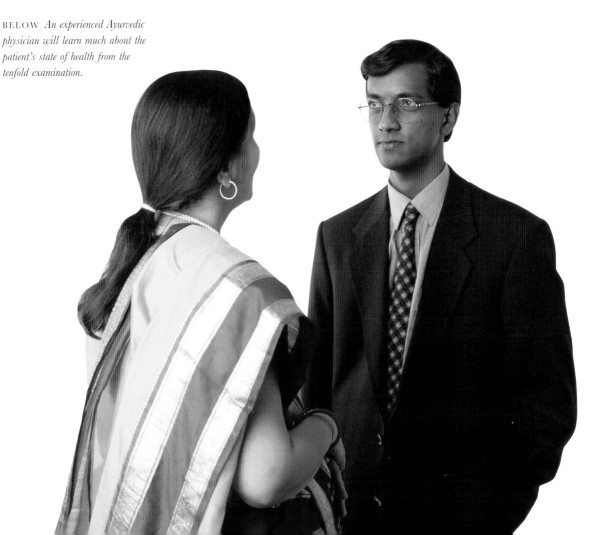

❋ **Adaptability** (satmya)

The term satmya means the substances that are normal to the body. This refers to two types of people. The first type is strong, tolerant of difficulties, and can digest all types of food such as ghee, milk, oil, meat juice, and all six types of rasa (taste). The second type of person is generally weak and non-adjusting and can tolerate only a few foods and only one of the rasas.

❋ **Psychic constitution** (sattva)

The sattva here refers to the mind, which is the controller of the body in contact with the atma, or soul. Depending upon the degree of strength, the sattva is considered to be high, moderate, or low. Accordingly people have three types of psychic constitution. The psyche is possessed of three attributes: sattva, rajas, and tamas. Those people with a predominance of sattva guna possess high psychic strength; those with a predominance of rajas guna possess moderate psychic strength; and lastly, those with a predominance of tamas guna possess low psychic strength.

❋ **Digestive capacity** (ahara sakti)

The individual's capacity for taking food has to be judged from his or her capacity to ingest and digest food substances.

❋ **Capacity for exercise** (vyayama sakti)

Capacity for exercise is assessed by the capacity for work, which is either low, moderate, or high.

❋ **Age** (vaya)

Ayurveda lays stress on your age, which has to be considered during clinical examination as there are a number of diseases and doshas that are prevalent at a certain age. Age gives vital clues for the diagnosis and treatment. Age is broadly divided into childhood, middle age, and old age.

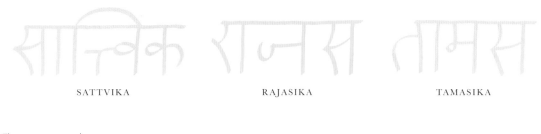

SATTVIKA   RAJASIKA   TAMASIKA

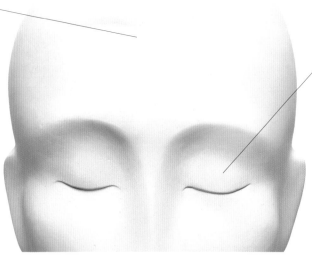

The sattva controls the body and has contact with the soul.

A predominance of sattva guna gives high psychic strength.

RIGHT *The psyche is made up of three gunas — sattva, rajas, and tamas — that determine your psychic constitution.*

MANASA PRAKRTI

❖ A sattvika person is kind, benevolent, intelligent, scholarly, courageous, bold, a believer in God, religious, and truthful.

❖ A rajasika person is impatient, egoistic, anxious for self-respect, ruthless, full of anger, indulges in excessive sex, and travels without any purpose.

❖ A tamasika type is irreligious, full of anxiety, lacking in intelligence, ignorant, ill-tempered, lazy, lethargic, and resorts to excessive sleep and sedentary habits.

Tamasika and rajasika qualities may seem completely obnoxious and you may wonder as to how two-thirds of humanity may fit into these categories. These particular descriptions are taken from the classical texts and reflect the intolerance of the divine sages toward human weaknesses. To them, only the sattvika nature was acceptable, and all those with human failings should resort to intense spiritual practice to transcend the illusion of wordly existence.

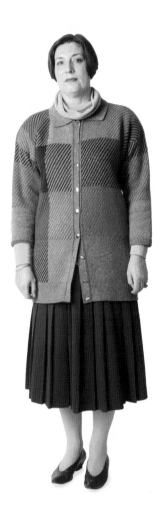 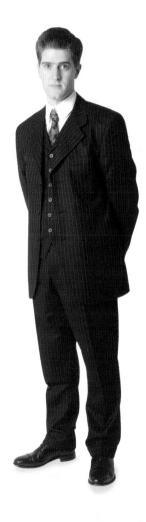 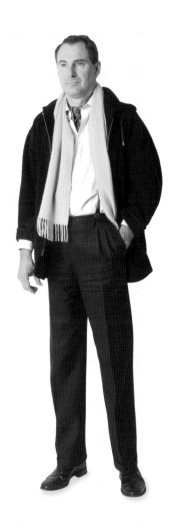

ABOVE *Giselle, a sattvika type, is compassionate, hard-working, and incapable of lying.*

ABOVE *James, an executive, is a rajasika individual. He is ambitious, shrewd, and action-orientated.*

ABOVE *François, an artist, is tamasika in character. He is unconventional and rebellious.*

The Eightfold Examination

The eightfold examination (astavidha pariksha) includes the examination of your pulse (nadi), tongue (jihva), voice (sabda), skin (sparsa), vision (drka), general appearance (akrti), urine (mutra), and stool (mala). This gives a fair idea of the nature of the illness and your general condition.

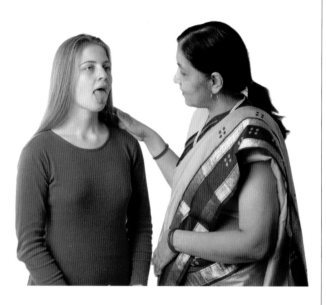

ABOVE *The general color and surface texture of the tongue provide an Ayurvedic physician with important indications about the patient's doshas and digestive system.*

◈ **Examination of the pulse** (nadi pariksha)
The pulse, or nadi, is examined for its normal and abnormal state. This is generally done at the root of the thumb by examining the radial artery pulse. Normally the pulse is neither very slow nor very rapid, and is regular and strong. When the pulse is afflicted by vata (vata nadi), it takes an irregular or zigzag course. When afflicted by pitta, it has a jumping motion, like that of a frog. When it is afflicted by kapha, the pulse is slow and moves like a swan. The characteristics of a combined doshic pulse are mixed.

There are a number of other factors mentioned in Ayurvedic texts linked to the pulse that are related to the specific condition.

◈ **Examination of the tongue** (jihva pariksha)
The tongue is assessed through its doshic state. When aggravated by vata it is dry, rough, and cracked. When aggravated by pitta the tongue becomes red and hot, and there is a burning sensation. Kapha makes it wet, slimy, and coated. The state of the digestive system is also assessed by the condition of the tongue.

◈ **Examination of the voice** (sabda pariksha)
When the doshas are balanced, the voice will be healthy and natural. When kapha is aggravated, the voice will be heavy; a voice afflicted by pitta will be cracked; and a voice aggravated by vata will be hoarse and rough.

◈ **Examination of the skin** (sparsa pariksha)
Palpation is an important method of clinical examination, including examination of the skin. It is also used for assessing the state of the organs and tissues. The doshic influence on the skin is also checked. When vata is aggravated, the temperature is below normal and the skin is coarse and rough. When pitta is aggravated, the temperature is quite high. Aggravated kapha makes the skin cold and wet.

◈ **Examination of the eye** (drka pariksha)
When there is aggravation of vata, the eyes are sunken, dry, and reddish brown in color. When there is aggravation of pitta, the eyes are red, yellow, or green, and there is a burning sensation and photophobia. Aggravated kapha makes the eyes wet and watery, and there is heaviness of the eyelids.

◈ **Examination of general appearance** (akrti pariksha)
The doshic influence reflects on the face of the patient and gives much knowledge about the basic constitution and the nature of the disease or illness that the patient is experiencing.

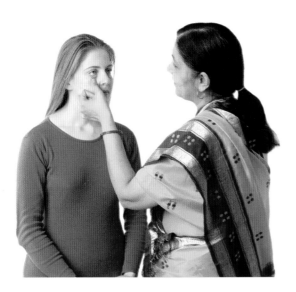

ABOVE *An examination of the eyes reveals changes in the color of the whites, as well as any discomfort or hyper-sensitivity that the patient may be feeling.*

BELOW *Both the speed and regularity of the pulse can be affected by doshic imbalances, and they also provide the physician with clues about particular conditions.*

❖ **Examination of urine** (mutra pariksha)

This is done by examining the urine sample as well as questioning the patient. The doshic influence may also be assessed. Another method of assessing the disease is the taila bindu pariksha, or putting a drop of oil into the sample of urine. It was traditionally believed that if the oil spread on the surface of the urine, the disease was curable and if it did not, it was thought difficult to cure. If the drop sank down, the disease was considered incurable.

❖ **Examination of stool** (mala pariksha)

When aggravated by vata, the stool is hard, dry, rough, and gray or ash in color. Aggravation by pitta makes it green or yellow in color and liquid. When aggravated by kapha, the stool is white, and mixed with mucus. Sama and nirama help to determine the state of digestion. If this is normal (nirama), the stool is neither hard nor watery and normally floats in the water. If digestion and absorption of food are poor (sama), the stool is foul-smelling and sinks in water. This may also give us a clue to any of the underlying gastrointestinal diseases.

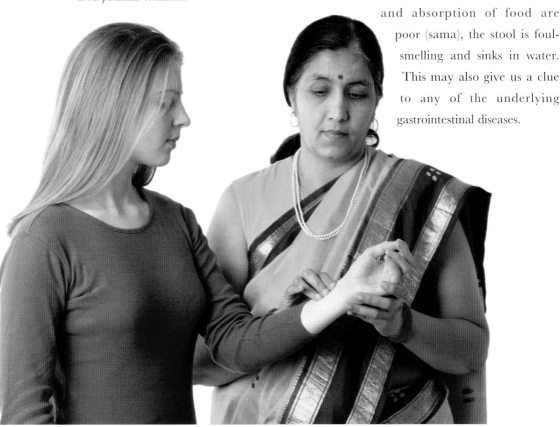

Classifying Diseases

IN AYURVEDIC medicine, diseases may be classified according to their effect (curable or incurable); on the basis of their intensity (mild or severe); according to whether mind or body is affected; according to their cause (endogenous or exogenous); and according to the nature of therapy required (medical or surgical).

Another way of classifying diseases is:

❁ Clinical classification according to the predominant doshas

❁ Classification according to the sites in the body, such as diseases of the eyes, ears, head

❁ Classification according to main symptoms

❁ Classification according to the morbid condition of structures of the body

❁ Classification according to the change of color of the body

❁ Classification according to origin (this is the most important method of classification)

A good physician will first assess the prognosis of a disease by the potential to cure it with all the means at his or her command and communicate the finding to the patient in gentle terms.

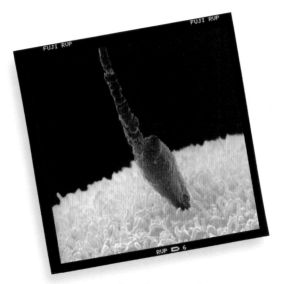

ABOVE *Some diseases, may be due to defects of the father's sperm or the mother's ovum.*

SEVENFOLD SYSTEM

In Ayurveda, diseases may also be classified under the sevenfold system.

They are as follows:

✦ Adibalapravritta (*genetic*)
✦ Janmabalapravritta (*congenital*)
✦ Doshabalapravritta (*constitutional*)
✦ Sanghatabalapravritta (*traumatic*)
✦ Kalabalapravritta (*seasonal*)
✦ Daivabalapravritta (*infectious and spiritual*)
✦ Swabhavbalapravritta (*natural*)

GENETIC

Diseases of this category are usually due to defects inherent either in the father's sukra (sperm) or the mother's sonita (ovum). Sukra and sonita are the primary reproductive factors for the formation of new life. If the defect comes from the mother, it is known as matrja, and if it is from the father, it is known as pitrja. If any part of the reproductive element gets damaged, then the body part growing out of it becomes defective, which may show early or at any stage of life. Recent developments in Western medicine also emphasize the genetic aspects of disease.

An Ayurvedic researcher in India linked children's psychiatric problems to their mother's emotional state while pregnant. He found a strong correlation between the mother's prenatal anxiety and the child's psychiatric ailments. He called it Abhimanyu syndrome, linking it to the story of Arjuna's child who learned the art of warfare while in his mother's womb from Krishna's discussions with his father.

Unwholesome food, abnormal behavior, addiction of any type, and stressful situations are likely to alter the reproductive elements of male and female. The examples of disorders caused by such problems include the following:

- Kushta (obstinate skin diseases)
- Arsha (hemorrhoids)
- Meha (diabetes mellitus)
- Kshaya (tuberculosis)
- Svasa (asthma)

Asthma, hemorrhoids, gastric and duodenal ulcers, epilepsy, certain forms of mental disease, and hemophilia are a few of the diseases that are genetically determined.

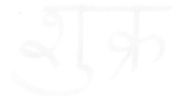

ABOVE *The Sanskrit for sukra, or sperm. If a genetic defect comes from the father, it is known as pitrja.*

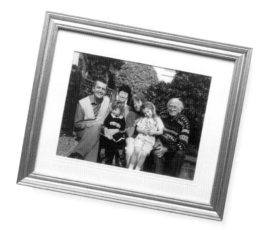

ABOVE *The Sanskrit for sonita, or ovum. If a genetic defect comes from the mother, it is known as matrja.*

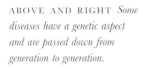

ABOVE AND RIGHT *Some diseases have a genetic aspect and are passed down from generation to generation.*

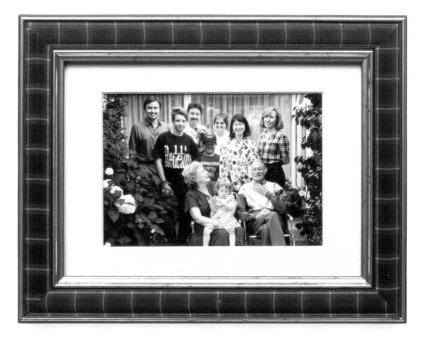

CONGENITAL

Congenital disorders are linked to errors in the diet or conduct of the mother during her pregnancy. They include congenital deafness, blindness, dumbness, nasal voice, and dwarfism. There are two types: rasakrita (nutritional disorder) and dauhrdya (ungratified desires or cravings of mother during the period of her pregnancy).

If a mother resorts to actions or eats food that tend to excite the vata dosha, this may lead to malformations and deformities such as kyphosis (hunchback), blindness, and dwarfism. The excitation of pitta can cause alopecia and yellowish pigmentation of the skin of the fetus, while excitation of kapha can result in albinism.

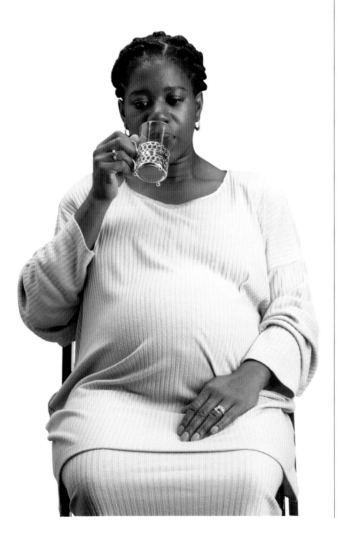

CONSTITUTIONAL

Diseases of this category are brought about by the action of any one of the tridoshas of the body, or by the two manasika doshas (mental doshas): rajas and tamas (*see* page 60). These may be disturbed by errors in diet, routine, conduct, or behavior. There are two types of constitutional disorders: sharirika (somatic) and manasika (psychic).

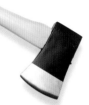

RIGHT *Trauma, which may be caused by sharp instruments, may be the cause of some diseases.*

TRAUMATIC

Disorders of this category include those that are caused by trauma (abhighata), which may be either external or internal. This includes injuries or blows inflicted by sharp instruments or caused by overstrain. Again, there are two main types: disorders caused by external injury and disorders caused by the bites of animals or poisonous insects.

SEASONAL DISEASES

This category includes diseases caused by changes in the weather such as heat or cold, humidity or dryness, rain or wind.

There are healthy changes that occur in our bodies due to normal traits of the season, and these are the usual adaptive reactions of the body. But there are diseases that result from the inability of the body to adapt itself to sudden and abnormal climatic change. For example, extreme cold may cause frostbite and rheumatic diseases, while high temperatures may cause burning sensations, sunstroke and fever.

LEFT *Incorrect diet or conduct while pregnant may cause congenital disorders in offspring.*

Examples include:
* Sexual contact
* Body contact
* Eating from the same dish
* Sleeping together in the same bed
* Using clothes, towels, and cosmetics of others

All of which lead to the spread of infection from one person to another.

NATURAL DISEASES

This category includes diseases that arise as a result of natural organic and functional changes in the body and mind such as senility, death, hunger, thirst, and sleep. These will happen even in people who have strictly adhered to the prescribed rules of health. These conditions are known as kalakrita. On the other hand if these changes occur in the body and mind prematurely, they are described as akalakrita, and are a result of living an unhealthy mode of life.

Diseases caused by the progress of age are also helped with Ayurvedic treatment. The Ayurvedic system has a strong armory of medicine and treatment for what is termed geriatric illnesses in the West, including rheumatism, arthritis, stroke, and its resultant paralysis.

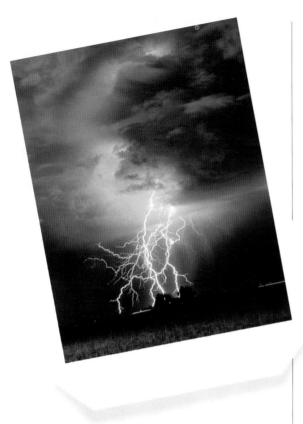

ABOVE *Acts of God, such as lightning, may cause spiritual diseases.*

INFECTIOUS AND SPIRITUAL

The diseases of this category are classified into two main groups:
* Illness due to acts of God (vidyudasanikrta) including such events as being struck by lightning, earthquakes, floods, etc
* Diseases due to influence of invisible malignant forces of nature (paisacakrta)

These are illnesses caused by other people's tantric activity. They have also been classified as:
* Diseases that assume the form of epidemic (samsargaja)
* Diseases that are merely accidental and confined to isolated incidences of a sporadic or endemic type (akasmika)

BELOW *Some diseases are caused by the malignant forces of nature.*

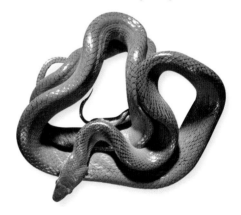

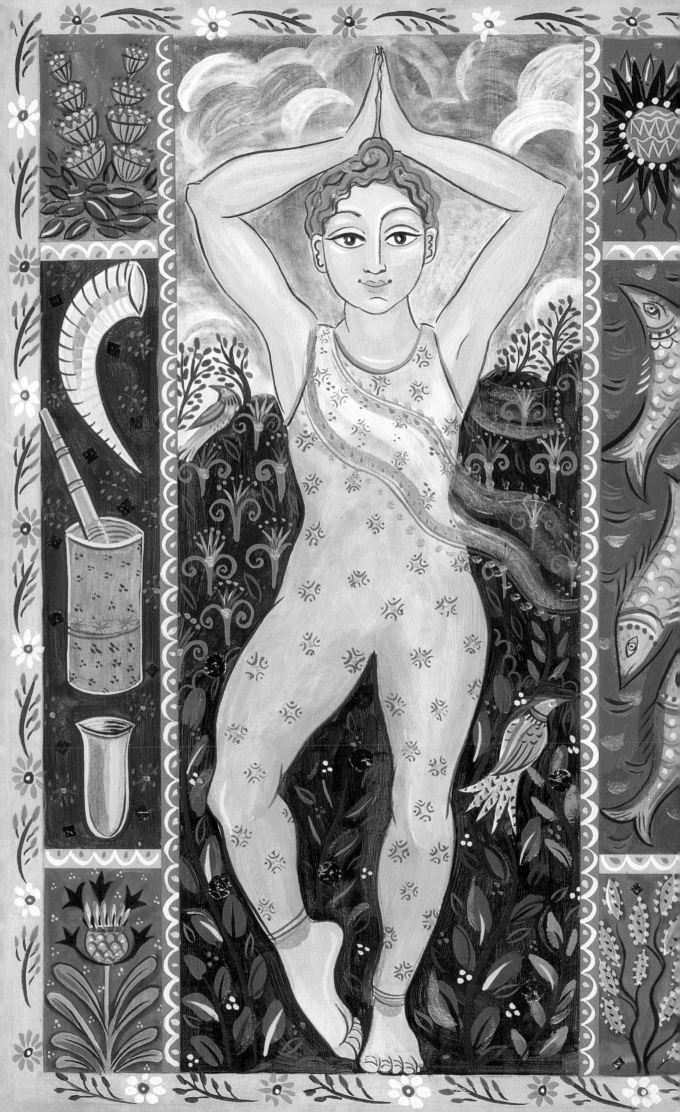

CHAPTER SEVEN

Treatment in Ayurveda

The heart *of Ayurveda is its many and varied forms of treatment for mind, body, and spirit. Ayurveda is holistic in every sense: prevention is as important as cure, and we must be aware of the right time to undertake treatment – a time that is right for the mind, body, and spirit. The techniques of Ayurveda are powerful, spanning the entire range of therapies from drugs, surgery, and nutrition to yoga, spiritual remedies, and astrology.*

What is Ayurvedic Treatment?

AYURVEDIC treatment consists of drugs (ausadha), diet (anna), and practices (vihara) prescribed jointly or separately, depending upon the disease, its prognosis, and the state of the patient. These various methods of treatment offer both preventive and curative forms of therapy to the patient. They aim at quickly reestablishing balance at the doshic level (*see* pages 46–59).

The physician, the drugs, the attendant (or nurse), and the patient are the four basic factors of treatment. The physician has the chief place because of his or her knowledge of disease, drugs, and in being the instructor of the nurse as well as of the patient.

The principles of therapeutics take into consideration two things: first, that drugs differ with respect to land, season, source, potency, and post-digestive effects; second, we all differ with respect to our bodies, constitution, age, vitality, digestive capacity, tolerance, and state of disease.

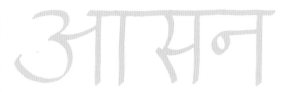

AUSADHA
The sanskrit word for drugs.

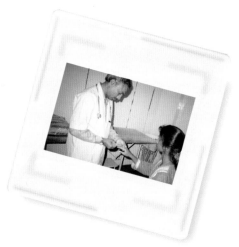

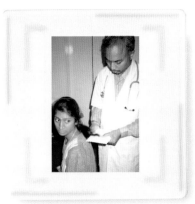

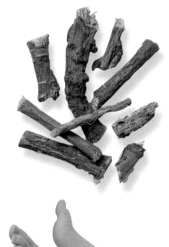

ABOVE *An examination of the skin and nails gives a general idea about the patient's health.*

TOP *Jethimade medicine used in Ayurvedic treatment.*

ABOVE *This Ayurvedic physician is examining his patient's hair for clues to her general state of health.*

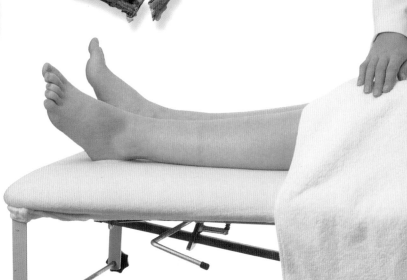

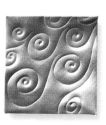

AIR

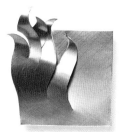

FIRE

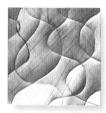

WATER

A nurse should feel affection and sympathy for his or her patient.

Cleanliness and purity of body is essential to good nursing.

TRIDOSHAS

The tridoshas (or three doshas) are the primary and essential factors of the human body that govern our entire physical structure and function. They are called vata, pitta, and kapha, and they are derived from the five basic eternal substances, the panchamahabhutas. Each dosha has a predominance of one of the five bhutas (*see* pages 46–59).

LEFT *Ayurvedic medicine comes in many forms, including powders, pastes, and tablets.*

Courage is necessary to aid recovery.

The patient must be able to describe his or her ailments without inhibition.

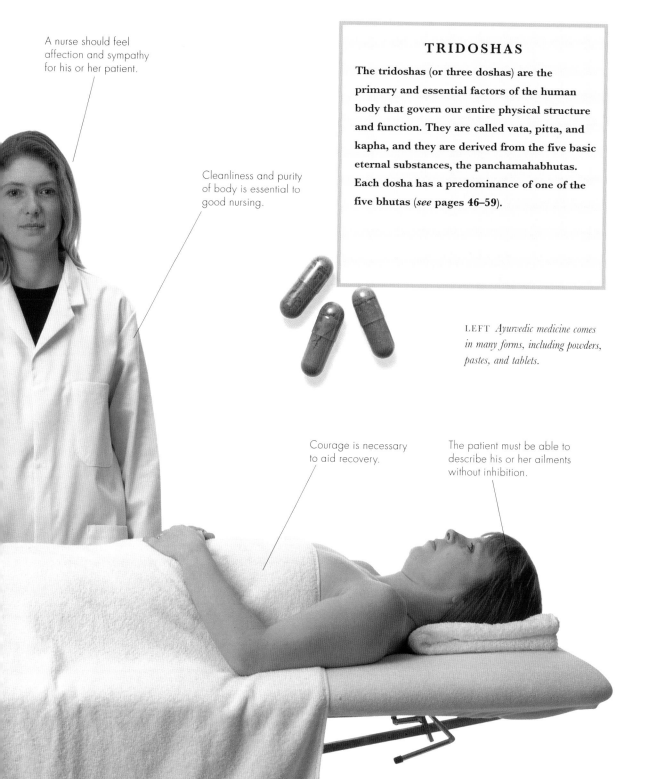

Four Pillars of Treatment

AYURVEDIC treatment aims not only to cure disease, but also to restore doshic equilibrium, promoting and preserving health, strength, and longevity.

Charaka writes that "all the efforts of the four pillars – physician, medicament, attendant, and the patient – possessed with the requisite qualities, for the revival of the equilibrium of the doshas in the event of their equilibrium being disturbed is termed as therapeutics."

Qualities of a good physician

❉ Excellence of knowledge and medical education
❉ Intense training in both the theory and practice of medicine and allied subjects, as well as having wide clinical experience
❉ Purity of body and mind

The Ayurvedic texts emphasize the qualities of each of these four pillars. Among them the physician occupies the most important place, as the person who cures disease and relieves suffering through his knowledge of various diseases and of drugs and other treatments, and as the instructor of the attendant (nurse) and the patient.

Qualities of good medication

❉ Abundance of supply
❉ Suitability
❉ Multiple form
❉ Potency

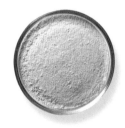

ABOVE *All medicines should be prepared in the correct way to ensure maximum efficiency.*

The herbs or minerals with which Ayurvedic drugs are prepared should have been grown in proper soil, gathered in the proper season, and collected with due regard to the principles laid down. They must also be stored and of course prepared (processed) suitably for the treatment of a particular disease.

There are patients who prefer taking drugs in paste form rather than as the juices of a drug. Similarly, there are certain diseases where medication must be given in a particular form (e.g., kvatha or decoction of drugs in treatment of fever). Therefore it is important that drugs are suitably prepared in various pharmaceutical dosage forms.

Qualities of a good nurse

❉ Knowledge of nursing
❉ Skill in their art
❉ Affection or sympathy for the patient to be treated
❉ Cleanliness and purity of body and mind

Qualities of a good patient

❉ Good memory
❉ Obedience to instructions
❉ Courage
❉ Ability to describe ailments (uninhibited expression)

ABOVE *Good training is essential to become a sympathetic and skillful nurse.*

LEFT *Obeying instructions is a very important part of Ayurvedic treatment for the patient.*

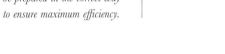

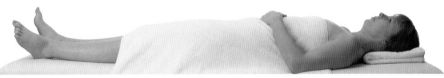

FORMS OF MEDICATION

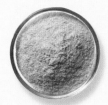

BALA

Coarsely ground bala is used to prepare decoctions, or kasahya.

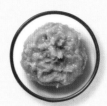

GULGUL THIKTHAKA GHRLTHAM

This medication is prepared in boiling ghee and is called a ghrta.

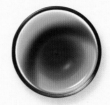

RHUMARTH

Rhumarth is a taila or oil, and is used in Ayurvedic massage.

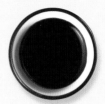

DASAMOOLA RASAYANUM

This form of medicine is called a avaleha.

Generally, Ayurvedic medicines are a combination of various plants selected on an historical and rational basis and are manufactured under different pharmaceutical processes. This is done in order to get not only their typical form, i.e., powder, expressed juice, decoction, etc., but also to modify and intensify their inherent properties.

Various pharmaceutical dosage forms are described in Ayurvedic texts:

❖ Svarasa – the expressed juice of any plant, squeezed from it, with or without the addition of water

❖ Kalka – a paste prepared by grinding the drugs, sometimes soaked, with water

❖ Kvath or Kasahya – a decoction. The drugs are powdered coarsely and then one part of the drug or drugs is placed in a vessel with four, eight, or sixteen parts of water. This is boiled, reduced to one quarter, filtered, and the decoction is separated

❖ Churna – a preparation of a drug or drugs in a fine or coarse powdered form

❖ Vati or Gutika – tablets or pills, made of various drugs, singly or in combination, separately powdered and then mixed in the required quantities

❖ Asava – a preparation for which drugs are soaked in liquids (mainly water), allowed to ferment for a specified period, and then filtered. To expedite fermentation, some fermentation agents are added

❖ Arishta – a preparation somewhat similar to Asava, involving fermentation. The decoction of various types are used for retaining their properties for a longer period

❖ Avaleha – this is a type of preparation that has a semisolid consistency and is prepared with the medium of sugar or jaggary as the case may be

❖ Taila – these are Ayurvedic oils. A special procedure is followed to prepare oils, involving a number of stages. The main ingredient is the type of oil or taila in which the other drugs are boiled

❖ Ghrta – a similar preparation to the taila, but the herbs or drugs are boiled in ghee instead of taila

❖ Lepa – a kind of paste used for external application and prepared with the help of water or any other liquid

❖ Bhasma – these are calcined products, prepared with various drugs being subjected to a high degree of heat

Four Forms of Treatment

KNOWLEDGE OF natural drugs has been a part of the healing art since people first began to treat illnesses. This developed from an ancient wisdom that used parts of plants and animals to concoct potions to eliminate pain, counteract disease, and control suffering. The history of Indian therapeutics can be traced to prehistoric times. The *Rig Veda,* which is the oldest book of human knowledge, describes plants and their actions. The *Atharva Veda* mentions the therapeutic uses of drugs in even greater detail. The authentic texts of Ayurveda – the *Charaka samhita* and *Sushruta samhita* – have broadly classified all medicinal substances into three groups: of vegetable origin, of animal origin, and of mineral or earth origin. The other texts of Ayurveda – *Astanga Hrdaya* and *Astanga Samgraha* by Vagbhatta – also deal with the materia medica of Ayurveda. A number of drugs used by the ancients are still employed in much the same manner by today's practitioners (although extraction, isolation, separation, and identification of the constituents of plant and animal drugs have occurred in relatively recent years). Nevertheless, the way in which many of these medicinal substances are employed today has hardly changed since ancient times.

Ayurveda treatment consists of four basic forms: medicine or drug therapy; panchakarma (the five systems of treatment); dietary regime; and the regulation of lifestyle. Ayurveda works in two fundamental ways – prevention and cure.

ABOVE *Preparing a traditional medicine in India.*

COMMON MEDICINES AND HERBS

Common Herbs for Panchakarma:

Madanphala *(Randia dumetorrum)*
Haritaki *(Terminalia chebula)*
Trivrt *(Operculina turpethum)*
Bala *(Sida cordifolia)*
Yastimadhu *(Glycerrhiza glabra)*
Rasna *(Pluchea lanceolata)*
Candana *(Santalum album)*
Amalaki *(Phyllanthus embelica)*

Common Medicines:

Narayan taila
Pancagavya ghrta
Candanadi taila
Dashamularishta
Pippalyasava
Triphala guggul
Anu taila
Kumara taila
Maharasnadi kashayam
Triphaladi kashayam
Amalakyadi churna

GUGGUL
*Used as an
anti-inflammatory.*

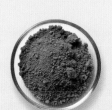

TALEESPATRADI
VATAKAH
*This preparation is used to
treat kapha-related diseases.*

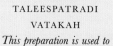

PASAMOOLA RISHTUM
*An excellent general tonic,
that relieves fatigue.*

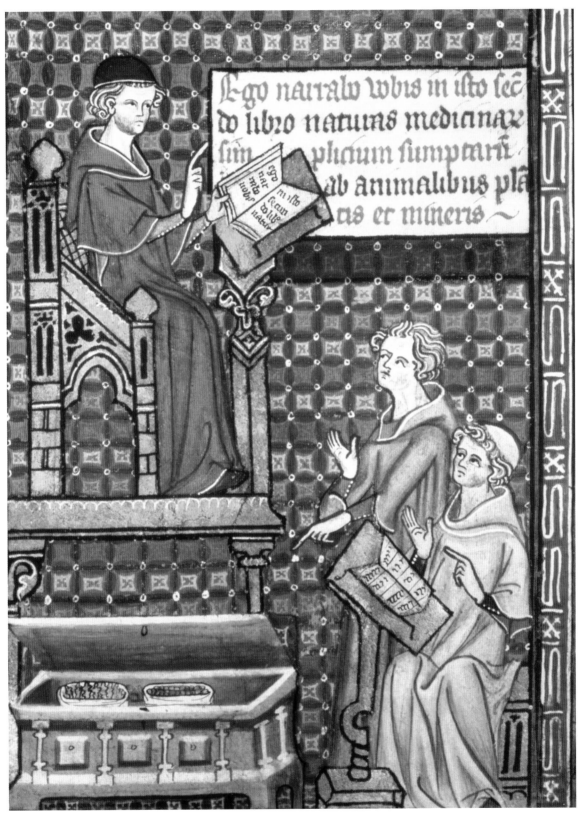

ABOVE *Knowledge of herbal medicines*
has a long tradition in many cultures.

Prevention versus Cure

PREVENTION

The preventive aspect of Indian medicine has three parts, namely personal hygiene, rejuvenation and virilification, and yoga.

Personal hygiene (svastha varta)

This is achieved through:

❋ Dinacharya (appropriate daily routine), including early morning rituals, baths, exercise, meals, and sleep (*see* pages 90–95).

❋ Ritucharya, or the regulations of life according to the seasons (*see* pages 96–99).

❋ Sadacara, or appropriate behavior (*see* page 178).

Rejuvenation (rasayana and vajikarana)

This involves:

❋ Special drugs to improve longevity, delay aging, impart immunity, develop body resistance, improve mental faculties, and add vitality and luster to the body.

Virilification (vajikarana)

Treatments include:

❋ Aphrodisiacs and fertility-improving agents.

Yoga

❋ Yoga practice keeps your body and mind in excellent condition and promotes well-being.

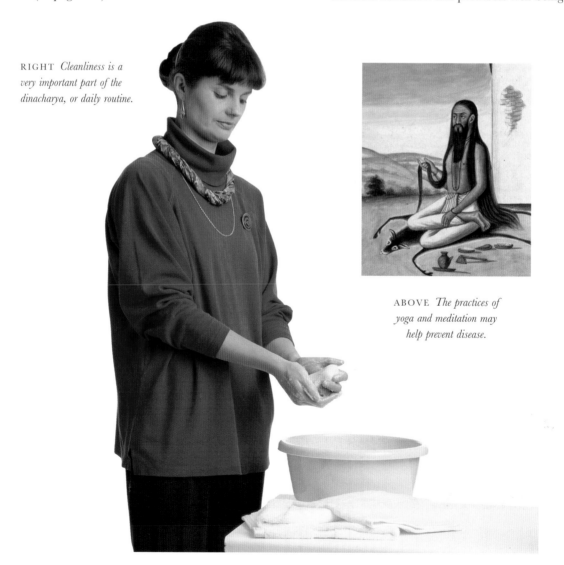

RIGHT *Cleanliness is a very important part of the dinacharya, or daily routine.*

ABOVE *The practices of yoga and meditation may help prevent disease.*

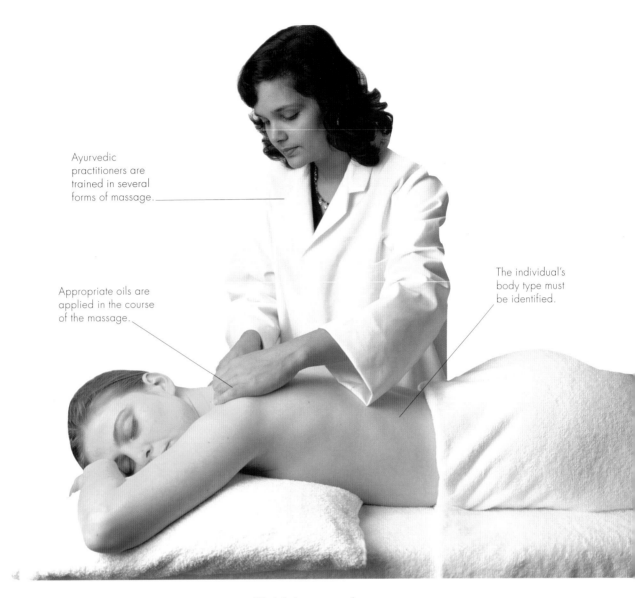

Ayurvedic practitioners are trained in several forms of massage.

Appropriate oils are applied in the course of the massage.

The individual's body type must be identified.

ABOVE *Whole body massage, using oils suited to the body type, forms an important part of external medicine.*

CURE

The curative aspect of Ayurvedic medicine consists of three parts, namely internal medicine (antati parimaijana); external medicine (vahir parimaijana); and surgical treatment (sastra pranidhana).

Internal medicine

Internal medicine consists of internal purification (samsodhana) and curative treatment (samsamana). Internal purification consists of the five ways of purification (emesis, purgation, enema, snuffing, and bloodletting), or panchakarma therapy. This is one of the most important elements of Ayurvedic treatment today, in addition to diet, lifestyle, meditation, and yogic practices.

External medicine

Used with internal medicine, external medicine includes: massage; oblations; application of pastes and powders; various gargles; and physiotherapy.

Surgical treatment

Surgical Ayurvedic treatment is rarely carried out today other than for minor conditions like fistula.

Combining Remedies

AYURVEDIC DRUGS

Drugs in the Ayurvedic system of medicine fall into three groups: vegetable products, animal products, and products of mineral origin.

VANASPATIS

OSADHI

VANASPATYA

VIRUDHA

> ### UNIQUE COMBINATIONS
>
> **Ayurvedic treatments consist of a combination of medicines. A patient being treated for a particular condition, say rheumatism, will normally be prescribed three to four medications, including an arishtam, a kashyam, tablets, and a massage oil. These medicines will vary according to the unique combination of a patient's individual doshas.**

❀ Vegetable products are further subdivided into four groups: trees or plants that produce fruits without visible flowers (vanaspatis); plants or trees that produce both fruits and flowers (vanaspatya); plants that die upon ripening of their fruits (osadhi); and creepers (virudha).

❀ Animal products used include honey, wax, fat (vanaspatis), and, at one time, coral.

❀ Drugs of mineral origin include metals like gold, silver, copper, and iron, as well as asphalt, lime, and gems.

These products are used singly or in the form of compounds.

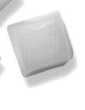

WAX

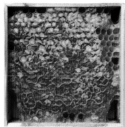

HONEY

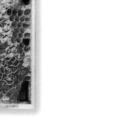

CORAL

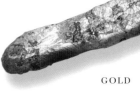

GOLD

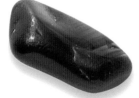

SAPPHIRE

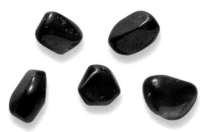

RUBIES

ABOVE *Ayurvedic medication comes from three main groups – vegetable, animal, and mineral.*

DRUG COMBINATIONS

On the subject of drug combination, Charaka wrote that "two or more drugs [together] exhibit… special properties that can never be produced by individual components because… they [either] act as a synergist and potentiate… [each other's] action or they antagonize some undesirable effects of some other desirable constituents."

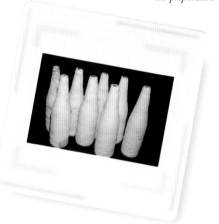

BELOW *Kachakupi bottles used for the preparation of rasayanas.*

Most Ayurvedic medicines are combinations of various drugs selected for their pharmacodynamic properties, including their doshic activity. The taste, actions, effects, potency, and specific actions of the drugs are important factors.

Depending upon these considerations, Ayurvedic drugs are manufactured and used for treatment in different forms, such as pastes (kalka), powders (churna), fresh juices (svarasa), decoction (kvatha), pills (vati), and medicated oils (tailas) – (*see* page 139 for details of forms).

These different pharmaceutical forms also help to modify and intensify the inherent properties of each drug.

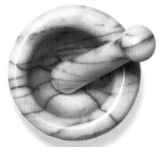

LEFT *Herbs are ground to make pastes or decoctions.*

COMMONLY USED MEDICINES

Common churnas (powders)

Asvagandhadi churna

Amalakyadi churna

Gangadhan churna

Common kvatha (decoctions)

Bilvadi kvath

Dasmula kvath

Goksuradi kvath

Haritakyadi kvath

Common vati (pills)

Gutika

Candraprabha vati

Kankayan gutika

Larangadi vati

Common avaleha (semisolid preparations)

Cyavanprash avaleha

Agastya haritaki avaleha

Kantakain avaleha

Kutajavleha

Common ghrta (ghee)

Amrta ghrta

Jatyadi ghrta

Kahyanaka ghrta

Common taila (oil preparations)

Arka taila

Bala taila

Chandanadi taila

Jatyadi taila

Common asava and arishta (fermented preparations)

Arjunarishta

Ashokarishta

Babbularishta

Drakshasava

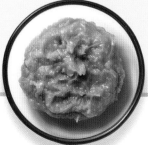

LEFT *Ghrtas are prepared by boiling herbs or drugs in ghee.*

The Correct Time For Treatment

AYURVEDIC treatments are similar to some modern Western medicines in that they are to be taken at particular times to improve absorption and minimize gastric irritation. For instance, some modern drugs are taken a half hour before meals. These include appetite-depressants (taken to reduce food intake) and anticholinergics (which decrease gastrointestinal motility). Other modern drugs, such as cimetidine, corticosteroids, and anti-inflammatory drugs, are taken with meals to prevent gastric irritation or to improve the absorption of lipid-soluble drugs.

Still other drugs are taken one hour before or two hours after a meal for more rapid absorption, such as oral antibiotics. There are also drugs that are best taken a half hour after meals to relieve gastric upset, such as antacids.

Dietetics (pathyapathya) are also important in Ayurvedic treatment, together with an adapted lifestyle, improvements to general conduct, and increased physical exercise. Emphasis is laid on avoiding incompatible diets, and there is a code called "tenfold ethics," which has been advocated while taking meals (dasa vidha ahara visesayatana).

ABOVE RIGHT *Some medications are best taken after food.*

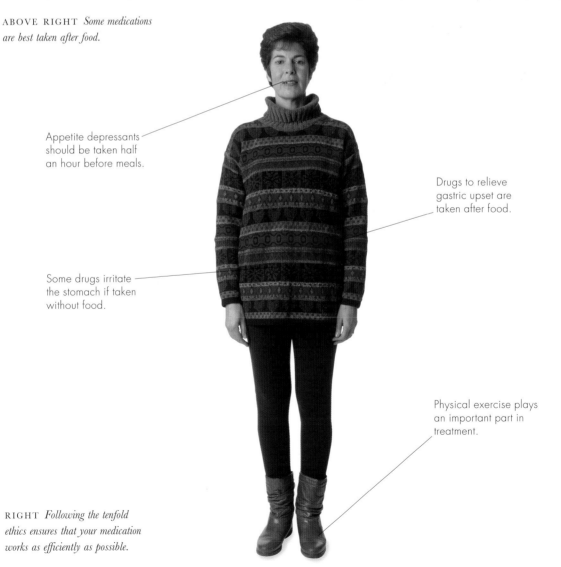

Appetite depressants should be taken half an hour before meals.

Drugs to relieve gastric upset are taken after food.

Some drugs irritate the stomach if taken without food.

Physical exercise plays an important part in treatment.

RIGHT *Following the tenfold ethics ensures that your medication works as efficiently as possible.*

TENFOLD ETHICS

Ayurveda describes ten proper occasions to take medicines. These relate to the timing of meals.

	Abhukta	on an empty stomach
	Pragbhukta	before a meal
	Adhobtukta	after a meal
	Antarabhukta	between meals
	Madhyabhukta	in the course of a meal
	Sabhukta	mixed with the meal
	Samudga	given at the beginning and at the end of the meal
	Muhurmuhu	repeatedly
	Grass	with every morsel of food
	Grasanter	with each alternate morsel of food

External Medicine

VAHIR PARIMARJANA, or external medicine, consists of massage, oblations, sudations, application of pastes and powders, different kinds of gargles, and other kinds of physiotherapeutic procedures. These can be used independently of, or simultaneously with, internal medicine. These treatments, like most physical therapies, are very popular with patients and the positive response to their use is growing.

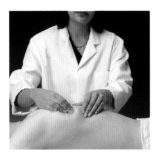

LEFT *Oil is always used with Ayurvedic massage.*

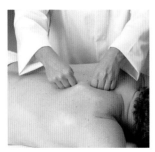

LEFT *Many strokes are used in Ayurvedic massage, including tapping and kneading.*

BELOW *Massage relaxes the patient and gives him a deep sense of well-being.*

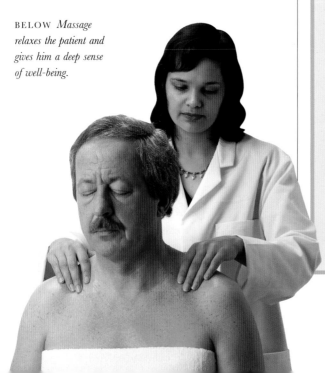

THREE BASIC TYPES OF AYURVEDIC MASSAGE

✤ Abhyanga – this is whole body massage with oil. Abhyanga is always given with different types of oils depending on the body type (i.e., vata, pitta, kapha, or a combination). The massage can be given by one or more masseurs, and is performed with a combination of strokes including tapping, kneading, rubbing, and squeezing. Abhyanga is always given prior to the herbal sauna. It is very beneficial for general rejuvenation, skin and musculoskeletal conditioning or problems such as obesity, body aches, and pain.

✤ Pizzichil – is a very specialized form of massage that involves the continuous dripping of oil onto the body of the patient from pieces of cloth dipped in oil, as the masseur massages the body with gentle strokes. It normally requires four people, two to squeeze the oil on the patient, and two to perform the massage. It must be done under medical supervision. Pizzichil is normally prescribed for general health and rejuvenation, as well as rheumatic conditions and paralysis.

✤ Chavutti pizzichil – is the most complicated massage of all. The masseur literally hangs from the ceiling by hooks and carries out the massage with the soles of his or her feet. The purpose of this massage is to apply the pressure of the masseur's body very selectively in appropriate nerve centers (marma) and in the tissues and musculoskeletal structure of the patient. This form of massage allows the therapist to vary the pressure and reach over the patient. Chavutti pizzichil is done with one or more masseurs, and with two or more attendants periodically pouring oil over the patient. It is used for patients who need to condition their bodies for high performance or those with acute problems in the nervous system, but not for paralysis or stroke victims.

Cecile is now completely free of acne.

She uses an Ayurvedic face mask and cleanser to keep her complexion clear.

Cecile has a high pitta–kapha constitution that leaves her susceptible to acne.

TREATING A COMMON AILMENT WITH EXTERNAL AYURVEDIC MEDICINES

Acne is a very common teenage ailment but it also affects older people with pitta–kapha dominant temperament during periods of stress or illness.

Cecile is an 18-year-old French girl with a high pitta–kapha constitution. She has suffered from severe acne for almost six years and had tried a number of topical applications. She had been prescribed several courses of antibiotics by her physician, but her spots kept returning the moment she stopped taking the drugs. She was also becoming allergic to the topical applications.

Cecile was prescribed two simple external remedies: one was an Ayurvedic face mask, Eladic choornam, to cleanse her face, and the other an oil to apply after cleansing had taken place.

The powder prescribed, Eladic choornam, contains: *Abies webbana, Acacia senegal, Aquillaria agallocha, Caryophyllatum innophylum, Cedrus deodor, Cinnamomum tamala, Cinnamomum zeylanicum, Coleus zeylanicus, Commiphora mukul, Crocus sativus, Ipmoca pestigridis, Kaempferia galanga, Limnathemum nymphioides, Mesua terrea, Mrystica fragrans, Nardstachys jatamansi,* and *Saussurea lappa.*

The oil prescribed was Kumkumadi thailam, which contains saffron and other herbs. Kumkumadi thailam is a very effective remover of spots and blemishes as well. Within a period of four weeks, Cecile was free of her spots and had a clear skin. She kept to the treatment for a year without any side effects. Afterward she used it once a week to maintain a healthy skin. She is now free of acne and has a good complexion.

LEFT *Cecile, with a high pitta–kapha constitution, suffered from severe acne. She was prescribed antibiotics before taking Ayurvedic medicine.*

Surgery

THE ANCIENT SAGES Sushruta and Charaka both write about surgical treatments, but Sushruta lays special emphasis on surgery, which he describes as the first and foremost specialty. He sees surgery as the most valuable of the therapies because of its ability to produce instant relief by means of instruments and appliances. He describes many major abdominal operations and also details 101 kinds of blunt instruments and 21 kinds of sharp instruments for surgical use. Many of these instruments resemble those used in modern medicine today. For instance, the simhamukha swastika (lion-faced forceps) are the forerunners of the modern lion's forceps. Unlike ancient Western surgeons, who were often little more than butchers, the Ayurvedic surgeons had a great understanding of anatomy, physiology and therapeutics.

BELOW *Some of the many instruments used in Indian surgery.*

Traditional Ayurvedic surgical appliances include thread (also caustic-coated thread – or kshara sutra – used in operations of anal fistulas), twine for bandages of 14 types, abdominal binders, splints (made of bamboo and inner bark of trees), suture materials, and goat's gut.

Thirty-two surgical manoeuvres are described by Sushruta. They include:

- Nirghatana (extraction by moving to and fro)
- Peedana (pressing out)
- Aharana (pulling up)
- Darana (splitting)
- Chedana (incision)
- Bhedana (excision)
- Achusana (suction)
- Lekhana (dissection)
- Vyadhana (puncturing)
- Visravana (draining)
- Sivana (suturing)
- Eshyana (probing)
- Bhandana (binding)

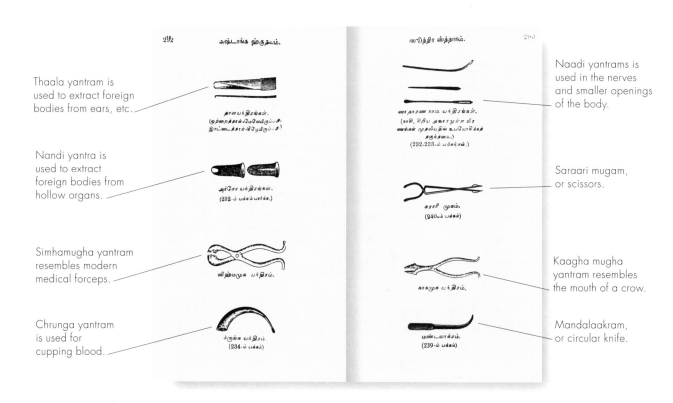

Thaala yantram is used to extract foreign bodies from ears, etc.

Nandi yantra is used to extract foreign bodies from hollow organs.

Simhamugha yantram resembles modern medical forceps.

Chrunga yantram is used for cupping blood.

Naadi yantrams is used in the nerves and smaller openings of the body.

Saraari mugam, or scissors.

Kaagha mugha yantram resembles the mouth of a crow.

Mandalaakram, or circular knife.

AYURVEDIC SURGERY

Shalya-tantra is the branch of Ayurveda that deals with ancient Indian surgery. Sushruta is the author of the classical text on surgery – *Sushruta samhita.*

Ayurvedic surgery in ancient India was related to the wars being fought in those days. In fact, Shalya-tantra means the text that deals with wounds inflicted by foreign bodies or arrows, and which require surgical intervention. This text gives a vivid description of various surgical procedures, including rhinoplasty and cesearean sections.

Descriptions of a large variety of sharp and blunt instruments, together with splints and bandages, are also found in Ayurvedic texts. It is interesting to note that some form or another of anesthesia was also used at that time to produce insensibility and also to restore the consciousness.

Important procedures like cauterization using ksaras and agni (alkali and high temperature) were used in those days. The techniques of cauterization, including thermal cautery, though bettered by present techniques, were well conceived and indicated an advanced understanding of the subject in those days.

Indian surgery's contribution to plastic surgery is also noteworthy. Rhinoplasty was first performed in ancient India and present-day surgeons can still learn from this work.

Surgery in Ayurveda, however, declined over time due to the efficacy of medical intervention and the absence of major wars. The lack of high-grade anesthetics was also a major reason that surgery did not advance beyond a certain point, as it is impossible to open up the body and perform long operations under quick-acting, low-grade anesthetics.

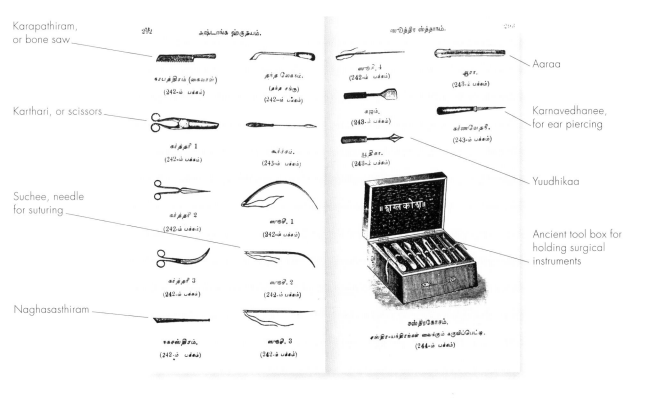

Karapathiram, or bone saw

Karthari, or scissors

Suchee, needle for suturing

Naghasasthiram

Aaraa

Karnavedhanee, for ear piercing

Yuudhikaa

Ancient tool box for holding surgical instruments

Psychotherapy

AYURVEDIC treatment also includes psychotherapy and spiritual therapy. This is known as satwavajaya.

Ayurveda takes a psychosomatic approach to diagnosis and treatment. The psychosomatic elements, and both physical and mental prakrti and doshas are identified in the development and presentation of different clinical conditions. Based on this concept, disease management includes restraining the mind from desire for unwholesome objects, and the cultivation of concentration, meditation, courage, and memory. A code of ethical conduct and treatments are also very important.

LEFT Consulting the Oracle, *a painting by Phung.*

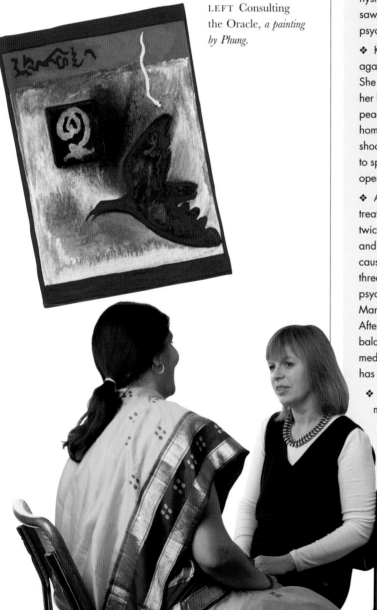

LEFT *A patient with psychiatric problems seeking advice from an Ayurvedic practitioner.*

PSYCHOTHERAPHY – A CASE STUDY

The primary cause of psychiatric ailments is the derangement of the vata or pitta doshas, or both. This case study of 29-year-old Henrietta illustrates the treatment systems used for psychiatric problems in Ayurveda. Henrietta is from a wealthy background. Her parents are leading members of London and country society, with a large house in the country.

❖ Henrietta was sent to boarding school at a very young age. A highly competitive girl, she started developing mild hysteria at school. She became jealous of her brother and developed a hatred for both her parents. Once, while returning to school after the vacation, she developed an attack of mild hysteria and was taken to see a psychiatrist. She saw him a few times, and was then sent to a private psychiatric nursing home.

❖ Kept in the nursing home for over three weeks against her will, Henrietta finally ran back home. She was happy here for the next three months, as her brother and sisters were away and she had a peaceful time. However, when her brother returned home for the summer, she tried to commit suicide by shooting herself. Severely wounded, Henrietta had to spend a month in hospital after an emergency operation.

❖ A close friend of her parents brought her to us for treatment. Henrietta was asked to perform meditation twice a day on a specific mantra to calm her mind and to pacify the excessive vata in the brain that was causing the disturbance. She was also prescribed three major Ayurvedic medicines commonly used for psychiatric problems. They were Saraswatharishtam, Manasamitra vatakam tablets, and Brahmi gritham. After two weeks we started performing dhara with bala and milk. Dhara is the continuous pouring of medication, including milk, onto the forehead. This has an effect of cooling the mind.

❖ After eight weeks of treatment, Henrietta has made a remarkable recovery and is now working in an art gallery in London.

RESTRAINING THE MIND FROM UNWHOLESOME OBJECTS

Unfortunately, with the explosion of media communications, a number of unwanted external stimuli intrude upon an individual in addition to those that he or she seeks. Even a number of the stimuli that people actually seek are in themselves unnecessary and perhaps harmful.

Some examples of unwanted stimuli include:

❖ Music and television in private and public spaces

❖ Noise pollution

❖ Public aggression, violence, or sexual abuse

Unnecessary stimuli often sought include:

❖ Exciting and violent horror films; pornography

❖ Continuous music through personal stereos

❖ Continuous watching of television programs

❖ Drinks, cigarettes, drugs

❖ Noisy and sexually arousing environments (night clubs, discotheques)

Although few involved in the spiritual or health-related fields will doubt the need to control the above types of excitement, the liberal-minded, as well as the fun-loving, will raise the question – whether life is worth anything if you cannot have some fun.

The answer will be to examine daily the nature of their attachment to such stimuli within themselves, through the process of reflection and analysis. The honest analysis of all such situations will show that there is some part of the self that craves excitement, an attempt to fill an emptiness born out of insecurity.

Further introspection and watching yourself in the act of enjoying the excitement will show that what it is doing is fulfilling some basic desire that is part of the fabric of your innermost being. What is called a vasana – a desire born of karma.

All those with addictive personalities carry with them unfulfilled desires from past lives and they are inexplicably attracted to them.

The trouble with all such unnecessary stimuli is their adverse effect on your body and your mind.

There is evidence to suggest that those who watch sexually explicit or violent films may want to enact them out in some way or the other, often leading to tragedy.

If you accept the need to control or eliminate these unwanted stimuli, how do you go about it? First you need to learn how to control or limit strongly desired excitement or stimuli through spiritual devices. This can be achieved by mental processes including:

❖ Watchful awareness of the self

❖ Catching the moments of desire

❖ Watching the desire and its fulfilment or its elimination by the will

❖ Watching the mind's and the heart's reaction both to fulfilment and to the elimination of desire

Other practices include:

❖ Meditation on a given mantra, or breathing as taught by a good teacher

❖ Yoga

❖ Prayer/puja/recitation of mantra

❖ Continuous practice of detachment

❖ Companionship of the spiritually inclined

❖ Reading noble and spiritual stories and books

❖ Visiting spiritual and holy places

Remember:

from desire comes feeling

from feeling comes thought

from thought arises action

from action comes habit

Understanding the pattern of your desire and your true reaction to its fulfilment or its denial is to know your own karma. Individuals who understand their karma come closer to true self-realization.

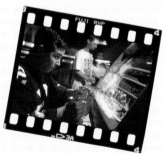

LEFT *Avoid exposing yourself to too much harmful stimuli, such as noisy amusement arcades.*

Panchakarma

PANCHAKARMA is the Sanskrit word for the five purificatory therapies used in Ayurveda. These procedures have great importance in the Ayurvedic system of medicine and are applied in almost all diseases – as discussed in the Ayurvedic classics. Another word for panchakarma is detoxification, an element of many modern therapies.

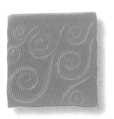
AIR

FIRE

Some passages of the *Rig Veda* text refer to the eradication of diseases through the nostrils, head, ears, tongue, and blood vessels, suggesting a knowledge of panchakarma in the Vedic period. The physicians of Mesopotamia used honey, milk, clarified butter, and oil to induce emesis, and purgation as treatment for pain in the abdomen.

These therapies are not only curative, but they are also widely used for the prevention of diseases based on sound classical Ayurvedic principles. Ayurveda considers the three doshas (vata, pitta, and kapha) to be primarily responsible for the production of different diseases when in an imbalanced state. These three doshas are brought to a balanced state with the help of the panchakarma measures, which include emesis (vamana); purgation (virecana); enema (vasti); nasal drops or snuffs (nasya); and bloodletting (raktamokshana).

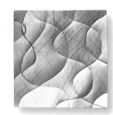
WATER

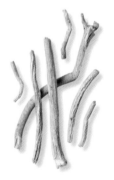
ASHWAGANDHA
This herb is used to give the body strength and boost energy.

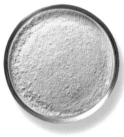
ASHWAGANDHA POWDER
The dried root of the herb is ground up to create the powdered form.

BELOW LEFT *Ayurvedic herbs in a variety of forms play an essential role in the preparatory massage and sauna that precedes panchakarma treatment.*

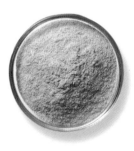
BALA
This powder is used in herbal saunas to treat rheumatic conditions.

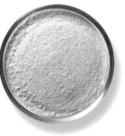
ASHWAGANDHA CAPSULES
In capsule form, this herb is used in rejuvenation therapy.

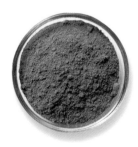
NIRGUNDI
Ayurvedic physicians use this herbal powder in saunas to relieve pain.

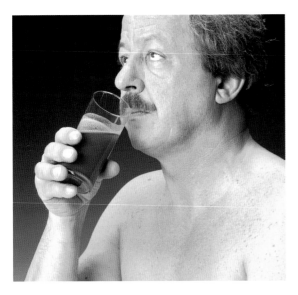

VIRECANA
*Virecana is achieved by drinking a
solution of Avipathi choornam or
similar medicine.*

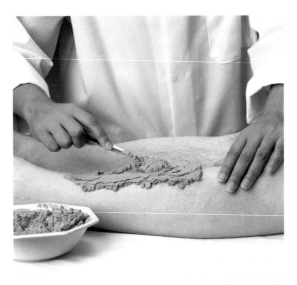

RAKTAMOKSHANA
*A paste is applied, and then
bloodletting is performed to purify
the blood.*

पंचकर्म

SANSKRIT FOR PANCHAKARMA

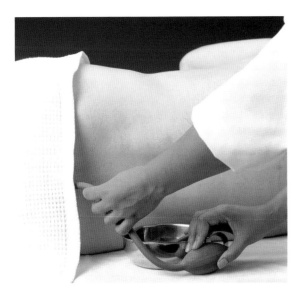

VASTI
*Vasti is the most effective treatment
for all conditions caused by
aggravated vata.*

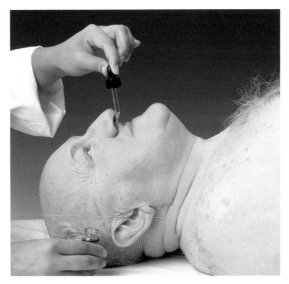

NASYA
*Nasya is the most effective therapy
for sinusitis, migraine, facial
paralysis, and other head problems.*

The Three Stages of Panchakarma

Panchakarma treatment has three main stages:

* **Poorva karma** includes preparatory measures such as the administration of oleation and formentation (snehana and swedana) before the main specific treatment
* **Pradhana karma** is the main treatment
* **Paschata karma** describes the measures employed after the main treatment, such as diet, medicines, and daily routine

The importance of poorva, pradhana, and paschata karmas in the prevention and cure of diseases has been recognized and emphatically stated in the Ayurvedic texts. Any attempt to administer panchakarma without proper preparation of the patient may not give the desired response and may also harm the body. Poorva, pradhana, and paschata karmas are essential in improving the body's own natural mechanisms. In all three stages, the patient must continue with the full treatment and not miss even a single day. The tendency to skip a part of the treatment due to inconvenience will reduce efficacy and can be harmful in serious conditions.

Diseases of the head are treated with Nasya therapy.

Emesis, or vomiting therapy helps eliminate kapha dosha.

The body is massaged with oil before the main panchakarma treatment is administered.

Your Ayurvedic physician may recommend a particular diet to follow after panchakarma.

Leeches may be applied to a patient's skin to suck impure blood from the body.

RIGHT *The panchakarma therapies are used in the treatment of most diseases in Ayurveda.*

Preparatory measures

(poorva karma)

According to Ayurvedic principles, the fivefold therapy should not be used until after the administration of oleation therapy (snehana) and fomentation therapy (swedana), which make your body soft and disintegrate the morbid doshas, so that they can be eliminated more easily from the subtle channels of circulation.

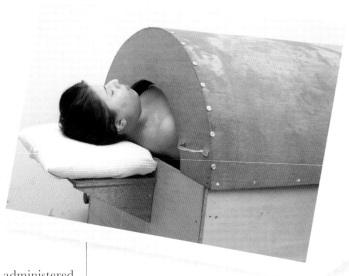

ABOVE *A herbal sauna is sometimes used to prepare the patient for panchakarma therapy.*

❖ Oleation therapy (snehana)

Oleation, or oil, therapy can be administered through different kinds of foods, or through enema and massage. The fats commonly used for oil therapy may be of vegetable origin, such as tailas, or of animal origin, such as ghee. These fats can be used singly or mixed with other drugs. Oil therapy takes from three to seven days, depending upon the individual's strength and response.

Improvement in digestion, lack of desire for oily substances, soft stools, and lightness of the body are the signs of adequately administered oil therapy.

Massage with oily substances and medicated herbs improves circulation and, by stimulating the system, speeds up the elimination of waste products. Such direct benefits – along with the physiological benefits of being comforted and cared for – can produce feelings of well-being that cannot be matched by modern drugs.

Once oleation therapy has taken effect, fomentation, or sweating, therapy should follow.

❖ Fomentation therapy (swedana)

Fomentation, or sweating, therapy follows oil therapy and should be given in a place free from exposure to excessive wind, and to a person whose last meal has been well digested.

Two types of swedana measures are described in the Ayurvedic texts. In one, external heat is required, while in the other no application of heat is required. The former includes poultices, decoctions, heated cloths, sand, and the steam of boiled medicated herbs. The latter includes physical exercise, covering oneself with thick blankets, hunger, and walking in the sun.

Once you are prepared by these poorva karmas, you are subjected to the panchakarma (fivefold therapies), depending upon your ailment and physical condition.

Both preparatory karmas and panchakarma treatment must be fully persevered with if they are to be effective. The patient should follow them with determination and not mix them half-heartedly with other "alternative therapies." This is why most panchakarma treatments in India are administered to patients in hospitals so that there is better control over patient behavior.

Main Panchakarma Therapies

Emesis therapy (Vamana)

In this process, the doshas are eliminated through the mouth by vomiting. According to Ayurveda, this is the best way to eliminate kapha dosha. Kapha is in the upper part of your body, and the elimination of doshas by the nearest route is an accepted principle. It is also known that if any dosha is eliminated from its chief place, the chances of any recurrence are very remote. The preparations used for this purpose are formulated in such a manner that their systemic action helps to eliminate harmful substances from the upper part of the body. Emesis therapy is administered with drugs suitable to the particular disease and condition of the patient. Common vehicles for the preparations used for this purpose are honey and rock salt.

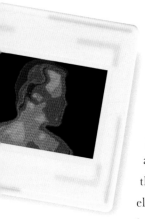

A feeling of cleanliness of the chest and stomach, lightness of the body, and timely passing of urine and stools are the signs of well administered emesis therapy. Physicians must take care to avoid over-administration as it could result in unconsciousness, blood in the vomit, weakness, and chest pain. At the same time, under-administration would result in not achieving the desired effect.

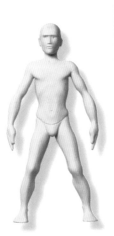

WARNING

On no account should you receive vamana or any other panchakarma treatment from anyone other than a qualified practitioner.
It is particularly important to observe the effects of vamana carefully as blood pressure can drop considerably if excess treatment is given.

USE OF VAMANA THERAPY

Vamana, or emesis therapy, is used for :

* Peenasa *(nasal diseases)*
* Kushtha *(leprosy and other skin diseases)*
* Navajvara *(acute fever)*
* Rajyakchma *(tuberculosis)*
* Kasa *(bronchitis)*
* Shvasa *(asthma)*
* Galagraha *(throat-choking)*
* Galaganda *(goiter)*
* Shleepada *(elephantiasis)*
* Prameha *(diabetes)*
* Mandagni *(poor digestion)*
* Hrillasa *(nausea)*
* Aruchi *(anorexia)*
* Avipaka *(dyspepsia)*
* Apachee *(lymphadenitis, or inflammation of the lymph glands)*
* Granthi *(nodes)*
* Apasmara *(epilepsy)*
* Unmada *(insanity)*
* Shopha *(edema)*
* Pandu *(anemia)*
* Stanya dushti *(poor supply of breast milk)*
* Arbuda *(tumors)*
* Medoroga *(obesity)*
* Hridroga *(heart disease)*
* Vidradhi *(abscess)*
* Putinasa *(rhinitis)*
* Kantha-paka *(pharyngitis)*
* Karna-srava *(discharge from the ear)*
* Adhijihvaka *(pangeutis)*
* Galasundika *(tonsillitis)*

ABOVE LEFT *Tumors are treated with vamana therapy in the Ayurveda system of medicine.*

CASE STUDY

Francis is a 40-year-old sales manager. He has been complaining of frequent coughs and colds, sometimes leading to breathlessness. He also suffers from throat pain and a hoarse voice when the condition is acute, as well as nausea, tiredness, and loss of appetite. Francis smokes about 20 cigarettes a day, and he has gained weight in the last year. No family history of asthma or other related respiratory diseases could be traced.

❖ The eightfold physical examination revealed a case of kapha aggravation and Francis was advised to make several lifestyle changes. He should ensure that he has adequate rest, and should stop smoking. When he is traveling on business, he should try to avoid exposure to hot and humid places. Exercises to control his weight gain should be performed, and he should practice meditation to control his anxiety and stress.

❖ Francis was also advised to follow a kapha-pacifying diet, and to avoid sweet and fatty foods. Easily digestible food should be taken regularly.

❖ The Ayurvedic medicines Lavangadi bati and Kantakaryavleha were prescribed to control his symptoms of aggravated kapha.

❖ Thereafter a regimen of vamana was administered. After preparation with snehana and swedana, vamana therapy was given using the vehicle of honey.

❖ Francis was then allowed to vomit without straining. As soon as he felt cleanliness and lightness in the body, the vamana therapy was stopped.

❖ He was then asked to rest and follow the post-emesis therapy regimen to get the full beneficial effects of the treatment.

❖ It has been a year since Francis' treatment and he has had no recurrence of the problems that he experienced before the treatment.

RIGHT *A change in lifestyle and vamana therapy helped Francis with his respiratory problems.*

Purgation therapy (Virecana)

Ayurvedic purgation therapy, or virecana, aims to eliminate doshas that cannot be removed by emesis or through other channels such as the kidneys, lungs, and sweat glands. This process of elimination of doshas is primarily from the anal region. It is a systemic therapy for the elimination of pitta dosha, pitta connected with kapha, and for kapha dosha situated at the site of pitta. A mild form of virecana is also indicated for the treatment of vata dosha, thus showing the wide scope of virecana therapy among all the therapies of panchakarma. It may be given three days after emesis therapy, or given directly when emesis is not indicated. But it must be practiced only after poorva karma (oil and sweating therapies) has been administered.

Purgation therapy is indicated for many conditions, including fever, skin diseases, bleeding from upper channels of the body, such as the mouth and nose, piles, worms, gout, vaginal diseases, anal fistulas, anemia, glandular swellings, and loss of appetite.

The virecana substances have been classified into three groups by Charaka. They include laxatives (sukha virecana), mild purgatives (mrdu virecana), and strong purgatives (teekshn virecana).

WARNING

Purgation therapy is not suitable for children, the elderly, or pregnant women, and should not be used for diseases like bleeding of the lower channels, weakness, debility, or diarrhea.

Enema therapy (vasti karma)

Vasti treatment, or enema, has an important place in panchakarma therapy and is considered the best treatment for deranged vata. Since vata is the force behind retention or elimination of various kinds, and the main cause of diseases of tissues and organs of the body, vasti is ideal for half of all ailments discussed in Ayurveda. Properly administered vasti helps to rejuvenate the body, provides strength and long life, and improves the complexion and the voice. Vasti therapy has been broadly classified into two types: oily enema therapy, and decoction enema therapy, depending upon the main ingredients used.

⁕ **Oily enema therapy**
(anuvasana vasti)

Vasti preparations containing oils or fats are used for this therapy. This is a complete treatment for diseases. Preparations used for oily enema therapy contain 2–4oz (50–100g) of oily substances. This type of enema is indicated when vata is excessively aggravated, there is excessive dryness of the body, and an

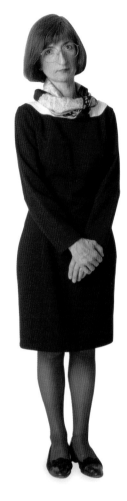

ABOVE *Vata-type constitutions benefit greatly from enema therapy.*

increased appetite for food. Oily enema does not produce any doshas in the body and can be given daily or on alternate days.

⁕ **Decoction enema therapy**
(asthapana vasti)

The type of vasti treatment in which decoction of the drugs is used to evacuate the doshas is called asthapana vasti, or decoction enema. Asthapana vasti returns the body's tissues to normal functioning. It is recommended for various nervous disorders, diseases of the gastrointestinal tract, loss of strength, muscular weakness, loss of appetite, urinary calculus, thirst, pain in the abdomen, fever, and headache.

The quantity of decoction used may vary from 24 to 40fl oz (700ml to 1.2l) depending on the intensity of the disease and the condition of the patient. The signs of well administered enema therapy are similar to those of purgation therapy (*see* page 159).

Oily and decoction enema therapy should be given in combination for the best possible results and should be planned with a view to the needs and physical condition of the individual patient.

⁕ **Enema through the urethra or vagina**
(uttara vasti)

This is a special type of enema given either through the male urethra, or through the vagina in women. It is recommended for men's genitourinary disorders, and for women's menstrual disorders. It is not suitable for people with diabetes. This type of vasti should only be used after proper preparation of the patient with snehana and swedana therapy.

WARNING

Oily enema therapy should not be used for some skin diseases, in fat and obese patients, for problems of the gastrointestinal tract such as indigestion, for loss of appetite, enlargement of liver and spleen, thirst, dyspnea, edema, or in states of grief or shock.

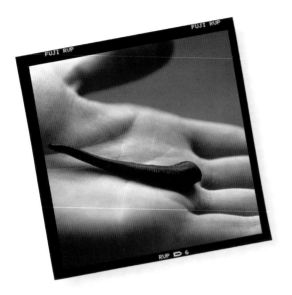

ABOVE *Nonpoisonous leeches are used in raktamokshana therapy to suck blood from the patient.*

BELOW *A paste made from turmeric and mustard powder is applied to the patient's body before bloodletting with leeches takes place.*

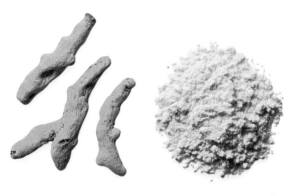

TURMERIC   MUSTARD POWDER

Bloodletting (raktamokshana)

Bloodletting is the fifth karma (procedure) of panchakarma therapy. Its main purpose is to eliminate some blood from the patient's body in order to tackle diseases caused by rakta and pitta.

Bloodletting is done either with metal instruments or by using other methods such as leeches or vegetable gourds.

Raktamokshana is indicated in all the diseases caused by an imbalance of rakta, such as obstinate skin diseases, tumors of certain types, gout, excessive sleepiness, alopecia, and hallucinations.

The mildest of all methods of extracting blood is the use of the nonpoisonous leech, or jalauka. The leech is applied to the patient's body after it has been purified with a powder or paste of turmeric and mustard. The leech sucks the impure blood just like a swan sucking milk from a mixture of milk and water.

Bloodletting with leeches is used in many parts of the world today, and its use is even making a comeback in Western medicine.

Bloodletting by metal or other instruments is a more severe form than that of leeches. This form is used when impure blood causes large absesses or enlargement of the spleen and liver. Instruments used for bloodletting include the horn of a cow as it has the properties of heat and sweetness, excellent for taking out blood vitiated by vata.

WARNING

Decoction enema therapy is not suitable for patients with excessive fat and/or those suffering from breathing difficulties, coughing, hiccups, low digestive capacity, piles, inflammatory conditions of the anus, vomiting, diarrhea, ascites (accumulation of fluid in the abdomen), or for pregnant women.

WARNING

Raktamokshana or bloodletting is not suitable for people suffering from general swelling of the limbs, debility, severe anemia, piles, fever, thirst, alcoholism, and unconsciousness, or for people who are old, fasting, or pregnant.

Severe migraines prevented the patient working efficiently.

The patient had been suffering from severe rhinitis for many years.

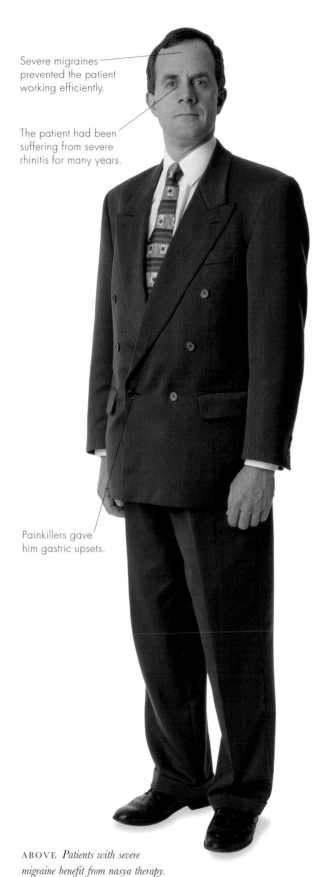

Painkillers gave him gastric upsets.

ABOVE *Patients with severe migraine benefit from nasya therapy.*

NASYA THERAPY

Richard has been suffering from allergic rhinitis and migraine headaches for over 20 years. He could cope with the rhinitis problem, but the migraine was excruciatingly painful and he found it impossible to work on the one or two days a week that he had the headaches. He had consulted a neurologist and an ENT surgeon, both of whom had found no major neurological or ENT problem.

An ENT surgeon had diagnosed a deviated nasal septum (a bent cartilage between the left and right nostril) and recommended minor surgery to correct the problem. The ENT surgeon believed that the deviated nasal septum was causing the allergic rhinitis. However, Richard did not want to undergo surgery. He was the managing director of a well-known international bank and could not afford days away from the office due to his insufferable migraines. His only relief was extremely strong pain-relievers and a half-hour lunchtime rest at the office. The pain-relievers gave him severe gastric upsets and it became a vicious cycle – the gastritis leading to headaches and vice versa.

In Ayurveda, migraine is called "suryavarta" as it follows the path of the sun, becoming worse at midday, and is due to tridosha kapa, i.e., the imbalance of all the three doshas in the sinus region.

The vata is obstructed by the deviated septum leading to kapha accumulation in the sinuses, and the pitta increases the feeling of pain along with the increase in the heat of the day.

The patient was given nasya therapy with Anu thailam. There are a number of ways of administering nasya depending on the severity of the illness. As the patient was strong and otherwise healthy, he was given marsa nasya, which has to be administered with a precise technique including:

❖ Pre-nasya massage with chosen oils

❖ A precise number of drops in each nostril depending upon the strength of disease

❖ The correct time and number of days

After nine days of nasya therapy, during which all the kapha from his sinuses were completely evacuated, the patient recovered fully. He has had no recurrence for the last three years.

Nasal drops (nasya therapy)

The use of medicines (medicated oils or powders) taken through the nostrils is known as nasya therapy. These medicated oils, powders, or drugs are for the treatment of head diseases and usually have an irritant effect on the lining of the nose.

Nasya therapy is recommended for diseases occurring above the collar bones, such as ear, nose, and throat, head and teeth problems, and for loss or premature graying of hair. It is particularly effective for sinusitis, migraine, or recurrent nasal congestion.

If nasya therapy is administered properly, the patient feels lightness in the head, and will sleep without disturbance. If the therapy has not been administered properly (for example through insufficient administration or over-administration of drugs), there may be excessive discharge from the nose and eyes, heaviness of the body and abnormal functioning of the sense organs.

ABOVE *Medicated oils applied through the nose benefit patients suffering from head diseases.*

WARNING

Nasya therapy is not suitable for patients suffering from fever of recent origin, indigestion, loss of consciousness, thirst, hunger, or grief, and it should not be used for pregnant women. Nor should nasal treatments be used for young children (under seven) or elderly people (over 80).

Paschata karma (aftercare)

This literally means the adoption of rehabilitative measures after the main treatment. In the present context of panchakarma it relates to such dietary measures and regimens as may be recommended to a patient who has successfully completed his panchakarma therapy.

Aftercare is a very important stage as after the removal of the doshas and internal cleansing with panchakarma, the digestive capacity of the individual must be restored. This is achieved through a properly planned diet and changes in lifestyle. By following an aftercare program, patients will reap the full benefits of panchakarma therapy.

Rasayana and vajikarana therapies (rejuvenation and virilification) can further improve your general health (*see* page 178).

AFTERCARE

Paschata karma, or aftercare, is very important for patients who undergo panchakarma. For each of the five treatments there are highly specialized aftercare techniques including completion of detoxification, special diet, the avoidance of specific activities, rest, and other special nursing care.

For example, after vamana therapy, the patient must rest in a room protected from wind. He is then given medicated smoke. The rest of the day should be spent free from loud speech, heavy foods, and daytime sleep. In the evening, he should be bathed in tepid water, and placed on a diet of red rice and liquids only. On the 15th day after vamana, the patient is given virecana therapy to clean out any remaining doshas.

Dietary Rules

As well as following a wholesome diet, everyone – both healthy and ill – should observe the following rules:

❋ Food should be warm, so that it helps in digestion and also with the downward passage of vata.

❋ Food should be oily, to stimulate digestion, to give strength to the body and sense faculties, and to improve the complexion.

❋ Food in the proper quantity promotes longevity, does not aggravate the doshas, and maintains the digestive capacity.

❋ Eat food only after digestion of your previous meal. If you eat before the previous meal has been digested, the undigested particles (rasa) get mixed up with the food taken afterward. This gives rise to indigestion, to impairment of digestive enzymes (fire), and to provocation of the three doshas.

If you eat after the digestion of your previous meal, it promotes proper digestion, appetite, proper manifestation of the natural urges for voiding, flatulence, urine and stool, and the downward passage of wind, and promotes longevity of the person.

If you sleep, take vigorous exercise, indulge in sexual activity, or even meditate immediately after eating, you will aggravate the pitta or vata doshas and eventually cause disease.

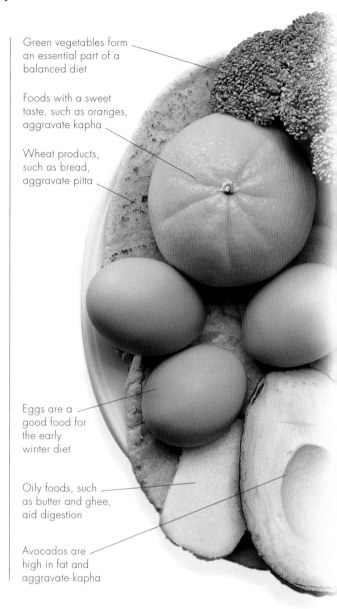

Green vegetables form an essential part of a balanced diet

Foods with a sweet taste, such as oranges, aggravate kapha

Wheat products, such as bread, aggravate pitta

Eggs are a good food for the early winter diet

Oily foods, such as butter and ghee, aid digestion

Avocados are high in fat and aggravate kapha

TASTES AND THE DOSHAS

	AGGRAVATING TASTES (RASAS)		ALLEVIATING TASTES (RASAS)	
Vata	Katu	(Pungent)	Madhur	(Sweet)
	Tikta	(Bitter)	Amla	(Sour)
	Kashaya	(Astringent)	Lavana	(Saline)
Pitta	Katu	(Pungent)	Madhur	(Sweet)
	Amla	(Sour)	Tikta	(Bitter)
	Lavana	(Saline)	Kashaya	(Astringent)
Kapha	Madhur	(Sweet)	Katu	(Pungent)
	Amla	(Sour)	Tikta	(Bitter)
	Lavana	(Saline)	Kashaya	(Astringent)

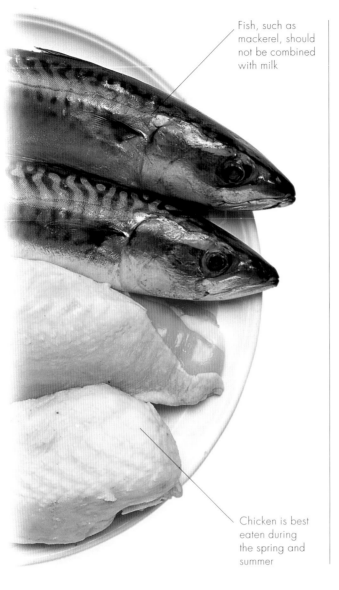

Fish, such as mackerel, should not be combined with milk

Chicken is best eaten during the spring and summer

* Eat food with no contradictory potencies. There are certain diseases that result from eating food with mutually contradictory potencies, so you should avoid such combinations. For instance garlic and milk, fish and milk, and honey with hot water do not make good combinations.

* Eating food at the proper place and at the right time helps to reduce emotional strain. Eating when you feel grief, anger, greed, envy, confusion, anxiety, or fear results in indigestion and imbalanced doshas.

* Do not eat in a hurry or carelessly as this means that food enters the wrong passage and gives rise to consequences that can cause serious complications.

* Do not eat too slowly as this will not give satisfaction and will impair digestion because of the irregular manner in which the enzymes come in contact with the food.

* Eat with concentration. Eating without awareness can lead to consequences similar to those that result from eating hurriedly. Avoid excessive talking and laughter while eating.

* Eat with self-confidence. It is advised that you eat food that is beneficial to your own constitution.

Knowledge of the benefits or otherwise of food is essential to good health.

ABOVE LEFT *Following a wholesome diet is an essential part of maintaining health and fighting disease.*

GLOSSARY

Vata	**Pitta**	**Kapha**
Vata is a Sanskrit word meaning "to move," to enthuse. Vata forms the most important constituent of the tridoshic framework and has a predominance of space and air (akasha and vayu) mahabhutas.	Pitta is a Sanskrit word meaning "to heat," or "to burn." Pitta is responsible for all biochemical activities, including the production of heat. Pitta is comprised of fire and water (tejas and jala).	Kapha is a Sanskrit word meaning phlegm, but also "to embrace," or "to keep together." Kapha is responsible for the construction of the living body, and it is made up of the water and earth elements (jala and prthvi).

Yoga

YOGA IS A science as well as a method of achieving spiritual harmony through the control of mind and body. The asanas (yogic postures) and pranayama (breath control) are practices that not only help us to acquire perfect health, but also develop the inner force that enables us to withstand stressful situations with a calm and serene mind.

The tradition of yoga was born in India several thousand years ago. Its founders were the Rishis and Maharishis, great saints and sages. All the sacred books of India like the *Vedas,* the *Upanishads,* and the *Puranas* mention the great sages who arrived at the highest degree of knowledge through the discipline of yoga – while still carrying on their various occupations.

Yoga is an essential part of Ayurveda. Its meaning comes from the Sanskrit root "yuga," "to join" or "to unite," and indicates the total integration of the individual soul with the supreme or divine soul to obtain relief from pain and suffering. Charaka wrote that yoga is the means of salvation (moksa), which is the end of all miseries (vedana).

Yoga was developed independently as a system of philosophy by Patanjali, the writer of the oldest text book of yoga, the *Yoga Sutra.*

ABOVE *The purpose of yoga is to unite the body and the mind.*

The art of yoga (as described by Patanjali) is practiced through eight methods, which are yama (abstinence), niyama (observance), asana (posture), pranayama (regulation of breath), pratyaha (withdrawal of senses), dhyana (fixed attention), dharana (contemplation), and samadhi (absolute concentration).

Each of these methods in themselves is an independent yogic discipline. If practiced in steps, however, they are far superior. Here we will concentrate on only one aspect of yoga, the postures, or asanas.

The word asana means "sthira sukhamasanam" or "seating oneself in a comfortable position."

The asanas induce a sense of physical and mental relaxation. Some have been devised in such a manner that they can be practiced irrespective of age, sex, place, or climate, and without causing disturbance in your daily routine.

These yogic postures not only produce simple muscular actions, but they also rehabilitate the various vital organs.

Bear in mind, however, that your body must never be forced or fatigued while practicing these postures. Each posture should be carefully, slowly, patiently, and properly performed, otherwise the results will not be positive.

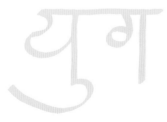

SANSKRIT FOR YUGA
Yuga means "to join," or "unite."

SANSKRIT FOR ASANA
Asana means "seating oneself in a comfortable yoga position."

CASE STUDY

Her stubborn personality may prevent a full recovery.

Amanda suffers from stiff shoulders.

Yoga helped overcome Amanda's stiffness and pain.

Amanda may suffer from arthritis of the knee if she does not give up skiing.

A manda is an American woman of 52 who carries herself gracefully and has a very dignified manner. She takes good care of herself but over the last few years has started developing stiff shoulders and knee joints. This was aggravated when she went skiing and her old skiing injuries became more painful.

❖ She was diagnosed as a vata–pitta individual and advised to avoid skiing as it would worsen her condition.

❖ She was prescribed Sahacharadi thailam, an external oil for massage on affected parts. She was asked to practice the following three yoga asanas five times every day – vrikshasana, uttanapadasana, and bhujangasana.

❖ Her pain subsided in a few days. Contrary to the advice she was given, she went for a skiing holiday. However, she still did not get back her pain. If she persists, as she may well do, due to her stubborn nature, it is very possible that she will get early arthritis of the knees and shoulders.

LEFT *Although yoga has helped Amanda with her problems, she needs to commit herself to a revised lifestyle if she is to remain pain free.*

Classic Yoga Postures

The five "common asanas" are padmasana (the lotus position), siddhasana (the posture of the adept), paschimottanasana (stretching of the back and hips), bhujangasana (the cobra position), and savasana (the complete relaxation posture).

The practice of asanas should ideally be followed by the pranayama. Pranayama is yogic breathing whereby the diaphragm, rather than the upper chest wall, is moving. The resultant breath is deep and oxygenates the lower portion of the lungs. Correct practice of pranayama under the teaching of a competent yoga teacher can dramatically reduce the incidence of asthma, bronchitis, sinus problems, and colds.

Pranayama is also a highly spiritual practice and is said literally to burn bad karma.

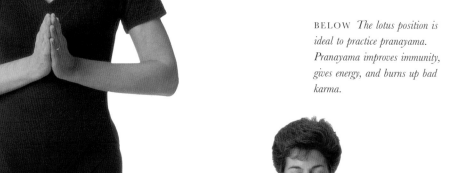

BELOW *The lotus position is ideal to practice pranayama. Pranayama improves immunity, gives energy, and burns up bad karma.*

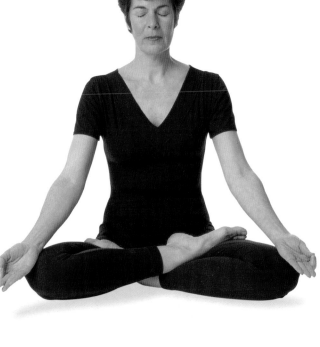

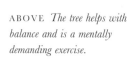

ABOVE *The tree helps with balance and is a mentally demanding exercise.*

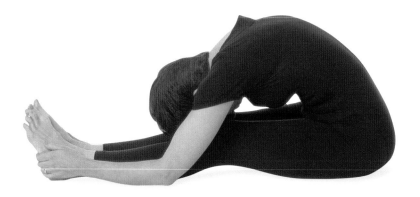

ABOVE *Paschimottanasana*
stretches the back and hips, and
helps make the spine more flexible.

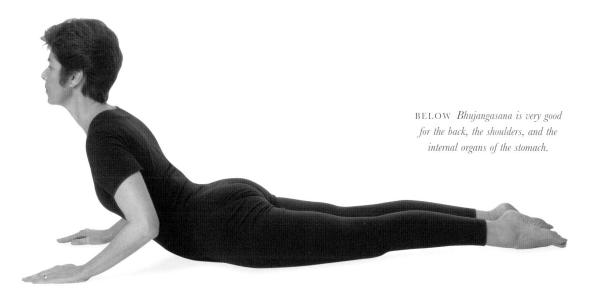

BELOW *Bhujangasana is very good*
for the back, the shoulders, and the
internal organs of the stomach.

BELOW *Savasana is the highest*
form of relaxation for the mind
and the body, and brings down
blood pressure.

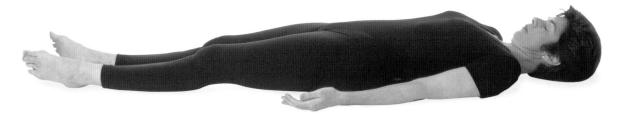

Astrology

As the living sage of astrology in India, Dr. B.V. Raman has written, "The influences of planets on human diseases appear with such persistence that it is impossible to ignore their effect." The sun and the moon provide the strongest influence on human healing, and their movements indicate changes not only in the seasons but also in human health and behavior.

According to Dr. Raman, "Crises in acute diseases are marked by the transiting moon and the most serious crises in any acute disease occur on the fourteenth day when the moon is in opposition to the day when the disease started."

ASTROLOGY AND DISEASE

Astrology – the study of planetary movements and their effects upon us – is a very important part of Ayurveda, and a good Ayurvedic practitioner will use Hindu astrology to help diagnose and treat disease.

The position of the natal moon (moon at birth) is also important in deciding the prakrti of the individual. According to the Indian system of astrology, nakshatras or lunar stars are very important for all aspects of human life, including marital relationships, career, character, mental behavior, and health.

Astrology also guides us to understand karmic causes of disease, and suggests nonmedicinal treatment like mantras, gems, and spiritual remedies. It also helps us to choose the right time for surgical treatment. Treatment carried out when the moon is in an unfavorable position, either for the surgeon, or for the patient, is certain to cause at least minor complications.

The 27 lunar stars of Hindu astrology, their houses of occupation, and how they influence the doshic prakrti of the individual is illustrated in the table below.

ABOVE *This eighteenth century Hindu astrological map shows the constellations.*

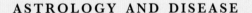

THE 27 STARS OF HINDU ASTROLOGY

VATA STAR	ZODIAC SIGN LOCATED IN	PITTA STAR	ZODIAC SIGN LOCATED IN	KAPHA STAR	ZODIAC SIGN LOCATED IN
Krittika	Aries/Taurus	Bharani	Aries	Aswini	Aries
Aslesha	Cancer	Rohini	Taurus	Mrigasira	Taurus/Gemini
Makha	Leo	Aridra	Gemini	Punarvasu	Gemini
Chitta	Virgo/Leo	Pubba	Leo	Pushyami	Cancer
Visakha	Libra/Scorpio	Uttara	Leo/Virgo	Hasta	Virgo
Jyeshta	Scorpio	Poorvashadha	Sagittarius	Swati	Libra
Moola	Sagittarius	Uttarashada	Sagittarius/Capricorn	Anuradha	Scorpio
Dhanishta	Capricorn	Poorvabhadra	Aquarius/Pisces	Sravana	Capricorn
Satabhisha	Aquarius	Uttarabhadra	Pisces	Revati	Pisces

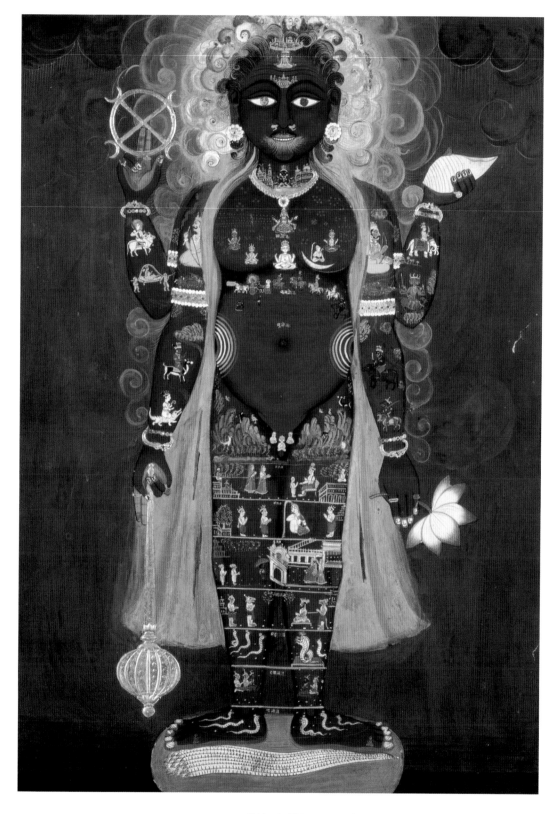

ABOVE *Krishna's Vishwarupa – the cosmic form of Krishna.*

How the Planets Cause Diseases

In addition to the moon, all planets have direct implications in causing different diseases. If you are suffering from a chronic ailment, your treatment should begin on days when the lunar star is one of the following (*see* page 170):

* Aswini
* Rohini
* Mrigasira
* Punarvasu
* Pushyami
* Uttara
* Uttarashada
* Uttarabhadra
* Hasta
* Chitta
* Swati
* Anuradha
* Sravana
* Dhanishta
* Satabhisha
* Revati

However, you should avoid starting treatment when the lunar star of the day is the same as your birth star and birth sign. Equally, if the moon is in the eighth house from your natal star, you should not begin treatment or have a major operation.

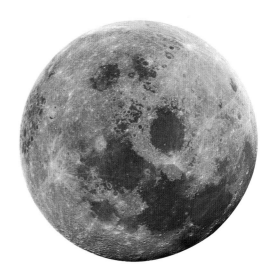

For example, if you are born in the star of Aswini in the sign of Aries, you should avoid commencing treatment for chronic ailments when the moon is in Aries or in Scorpio. Emergency treatment cannot be avoided, of course, at any time. The same also applies to surgical treatments. Major surgery should be avoided on these days, unless in a life-threatening situation. These are simple rules to follow but they can have significant benefits for the patient.

A notorious time for ailments for humans (it is thought even incarnated gods) is the period called sade sathi, or the seven-and-a-half-year period of Saturn when Saturn transits the 12th, 1st, and 2nd houses to the natal star. At such a time only prayers, remedial rituals, and the wearing of appropriate gems can be of some assistance.

Yet this period is a great educator of the soul, and we can evolve through our karmic cycles and emerge stronger at the end of the seven-and-a-half years if we spend at least some of this period in a spirit of soul-searching, prayer, and contemplation.

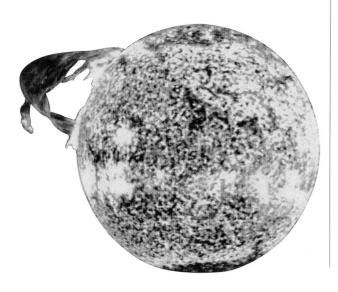

LEFT *The sun's effect is felt not only in the seasons, but in health and behavior.*

ABOVE *The influence of the moon is very important in assessing health problems and the right time for treatment.*

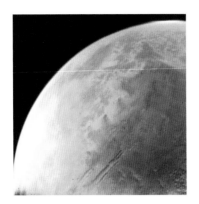

MARS
*Unfavorable Mars can cause
a variety of illnesses. Wearing
corals may help.*

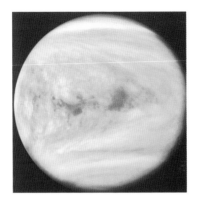

VENUS
*Venus may cause gynecological
and sexual diseases. Diamond is
the gem for Venus.*

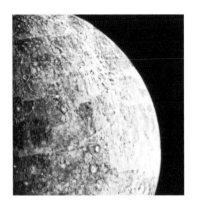

MERCURY
*Mercury is the cause of many
ailments. Emerald is the
stone for Mercury.*

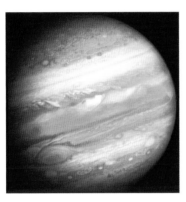

JUPITER
*Jupiter causes obesity and urinary
problems. Topaz is the stone
for this planet.*

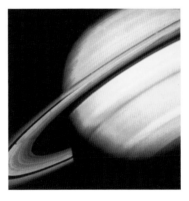

SATURN
*Saturn can cause a variety of
ailments and sorrow. Dark blue
sapphire is the stone for Saturn.*

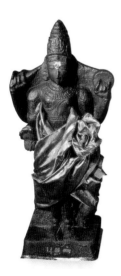
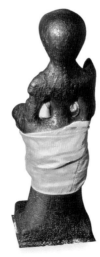
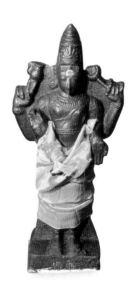

ABOVE *The planets represented in
deity form within a Hindu temple.*

How Gems can Prevent Disease

The wearing of specific gems helps us to reduce the impact of planetary afflictions on our bodies.

You should consult an astrologer or an expert Ayurvedic physician to select the right gem as this requires the casting of your individual horoscope as well as a clear understanding of the disease and the karmic patterns of the individual. The wrong gem can aggravate the condition and may cause you other problems.

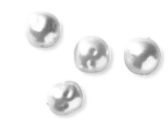

PEARL
Pearls are used to treat rheumatism, musculoskeletal problems, and bone diseases.

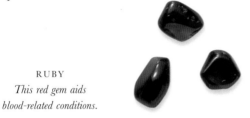

RUBY
This red gem aids blood-related conditions.

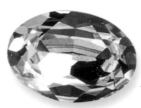

DIAMOND
Diamonds help treat urinary and gynecological problems.

THE APPROPRIATE GEMS FOR EACH DISEASE AND THEIR PLANETARY RULERS

DISEASE	GEM	PLANET
Rheumatism, musculoskeletal problems, and bone diseases	Red coral, emerald, pearl, dark blue sapphire, ruby	Mars, Mercury, moon, Saturn, sun
Digestive diseases, including diabetes	Red coral, white coral, emerald	Mars, Mercury
Diseases of the nervous system	Dark blue sapphire	Saturn, ketu
Psychological diseases, including hysteria	Emerald in the night, red coral in the day	Mercury, Mars, ketu
Skin diseases	White coral, yellow sapphire	Mars, Saturn, rahu
Urinary and gynecological problems	Pearl, diamond, red coral, yellow sapphire, emerald, topaz	moon, Venus, Mars, Saturn, Mercury, Jupiter
Dental problems	Sapphire, red coral	Saturn, Mars
Ear, nose, and throat problems	Yellow sapphire, white coral	Saturn, Mars
Blood-related problems	Dark blue sapphire, emerald, ruby	Saturn, Mercury, sun, rahu

Rahu and ketu are nodal points exactly opposite each other and are given the status of planets according to the Indian system of astrology. They are important indicators of spiritual and/or materialistic tendencies.

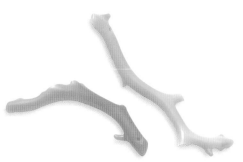

RED CORAL
*This precious material is ruled
by the red planet.*

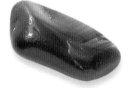

SAPPHIRE
*Muscular and nervous diseases are
eased by sapphires.*

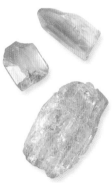

TOPAZ
*Topaz is ruled by the moon and
several planets.*

CASE STUDY

❖ The period of Saturn called sade sathi (seven-and-a-half-year period of Saturn) is notorious for the difficulties it inflicts on those under its influence. This is the period when Saturn transits over the 12th, 1st and 2nd houses to the natal moon. In other words, if the moon is in the sign of Capricorn at birth when Saturn moves through the sign of Sagittarius, Capricorn and Aquarius, it is a difficult period for the individual.

❖ Stephen's moon is in the sign of Sagittarius. During the transit of the moon through the sign of Scorpio, our patient started experiencing major problems, including family tragedies and personal illness.

❖ In addition to the appropriate treatments for his ailments, he was taught a specific, powerful mantra for the planet Saturn. He was asked to wear a dark blue sapphire ring in such a way that the stone actually touched his body at all times.

❖ He continued to have some difficulties and problems, but found that he could now cope with them, and many of the problems that had seemed insurmountable when they initially appeared, were overcome with the intense recitation of the mantra.

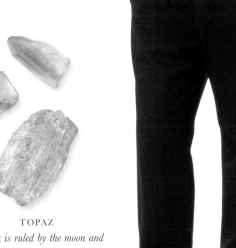

LEFT *Planetary influences can play a
major part in both family life and
personal health. Gems can counteract
these influences.*

Spiritual Remedies

PRAYERS, MANTRAS, and remedial rituals are an essential part of Ayurveda, particularly for serious and chronic ailments. All diseases are the product of individual karma. The only way to transcend your negative karma is through good actions, and the invocation of divine help through mantra and prayer. A good Ayurvedic physician should be able to guide you.

Mantra works even more miraculously than any medicine as it penetrates deep into the organs and tissues affected by disease, carrying out the necessary repair work without the aid of medicine.

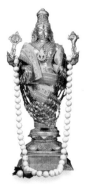

BALAJI

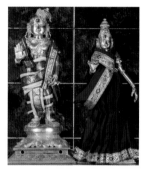

RADHA AND
KRISHNA

THE POWER OF PRAYER

In Hinduism, the two gods for healing are Vishnu and Shiva, particularly in their forms as Dhanwantari and Dakshinamurti. Other male deities worshipped for the cure of diseases are the sons of Shiva: Kartikeya, and Ganesha. The most powerful Hindu goddess worshipped for the cure of ailments is Durga, the consort of Shiva.

Vishnu, in his form as Krishna, also has great curative powers, particularly for conditions such as rheumatism. One of the most famous temples for the cure of rheumatism is the temple of Krishna in Guruvayoor in Kerala, India.

Melppatthur, the poet, was completely crippled by disease when he was taken in a stretcher to the temple of Guruvayoor. Lying on his bed for over 40 days, the poet composed his famous long poem, the "Narayaneeyam," in praise of Krishna. At the end of the last stanza he was able to get up, and after prostrating himself at the feet of the deity, he walked out of the temple, crying tears of joy.

Hinduism does not ever say that only the gods of its own pantheon should be worshipped. The true Hindu believes that any truly religious person should worship their own god or goddess sincerely and – most importantly – with humility and complete surrender. Thus, to a true Hindu, a true

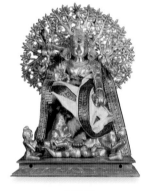

LORD
DAKSHINAMURTI

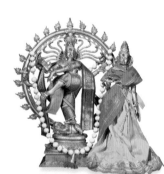

NATARAJA

Muslim is an equally noble soul and no religious person should dismiss another as a "fundamentalist" simply because they believe intensely in their god.

THE POWER OF MANTRA

There are very powerful mantras, yantras (geometric designs like the sri chakra), and other practices in Hinduism to heal disease and to protect yourself physically, spiritually, and psychically. But in all of these you must be instructed by a teacher.

Each deity has powerful bijamantras (seed syllable mantras), including "om," which should only be taught to you personally by your teacher. Any mantra not transmitted through a personal teacher is powerless and can mislead. But your surrender to your teacher and your humility before him is for

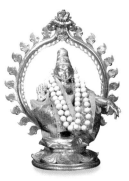

SHASTA

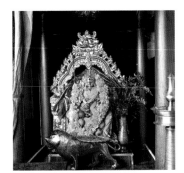

SRI DURGA

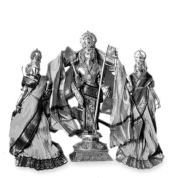

KARTHIKEYA

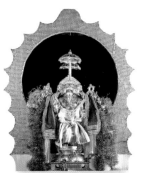

LORD GANAPATHY

your benefit and not for his ego. Yet there is no use in trying to repeat a mantra or worship a deity if your heart continues to whisper, "Oh! This is not right for me." In other words, your prayer or mantra must be intellectually and emotionally acceptable to you.

There is a current refrain in the West and even in India that all gurus and teachers of spirituality are frauds and charlatans only out to make money and seduce women. Disciples and seekers will always get the kind of guru they deserve. Those contaminated by material desires, ego, and power will inevitably find a similar teacher or cult figure as their inner vibrations on that level can only correspond to someone of a similar orientation. Very often disciples can corrupt such teachers and draw him down further to their own levels.

Until such egoism is rooted out, the suspicion of gurus will continue, and so will the inability of the spiritual seeker to find solace in this world of deep suffering and pain.

KRISHNA'S GAME

While this book was being written, a young South African girl of English origin walked straight into my office, without a prior appointment, seeking advice.

I asked her immediately if she was a Krishna devotee, because I felt something to that effect. She immediately said, "No, definitely not."

Then she described her journey through many books and a number of disciplines including Reiki, Rolfing, rebirthing, and herbalism. She said she was angry with her parents because rebirthing told her they were cruel to her. She began to cry. She said she was confused and wanted to die, to commit suicide.

I asked her why she did not throw away all her books, her practices, all her outward search, and turn only to God, and quoted the words of Krishna in the *Bhagavad Gita*, "Sarva dharma parityjya Mameka Saranam Vraja."

"Forget all your duties and take refuge in me." That she should find her own refuge in her own God.

She immediately retorted, "I was a Hare Krishna devotee for five years. Oh, they are mad."

I could only laugh at Krishna's game on his old devotee who had deserted him for the human kind!

When this was explained to her, the girl, who was undoubtedly a completely genuine seeker, immediately saw the connection and went away with something to think about, still in tears.

Rejuvenation and Virilification Therapy

REJUVENATION THERAPY

The treatment or chikitsa, as it is known in Ayurveda, seeks to achieve two objectives. Rejuvenation therapy, or rasayana, helps to promote and preserve health and longevity in the healthy, and to cure disease in the sick.

Rasayana is important in the ancient texts of Ayurveda, and Charaka wrote a complete chapter on this subject. Depending upon your age, individual constitution, adaptability, the condition of your sense organs, and your digestive capacity, a suitable rasayana agent is selected.

These rasayana drugs either improve your nutritional status, or improve your digestive capacity and metabolic activity:

❀ **Medhya rasayana** (for the intellect)

Rasayana drugs rejuvenate your body as well as your mind. A special category of rasayana drugs improve your medhya, or the intellect, memory, and willpower. These important drugs have a wide psychotropic action, and they include Brahmi, Jyotismati, Asvagandha, Sankhapuspi, and Vaca.

❀ **Naimittika rasayana** (for vitality)

Some rasayana drugs are prescribed to improve your vitality when you have a specific disease. For example:

❀ Jyotismati, Triphala (for eye disease)
❀ Arjuna, Salaparni (for heart disease)
❀ Lauha (for anemia)
❀ Haridra (for allergic diseases)
❀ Guggul (for obesity and lipid disorders)

VAJIKARANA THERAPY

Vajikarana therapy promotes fertility and virility in men. Vajikarana drugs are used as aphrodisiacs and fertility-improving agents. They can induce an immediate sense of pleasurable excitement, together with increased and fertile seminal secretions – even in an aging person. These drugs also bestow considerable sexual stamina.

In the ultimate sense, these drugs make possible the achievement of the man's desire for excellent offspring to carry forward his tradition and lineage. However, vajikarana therapy must be used with care to achieve the purpose of procreation. To abuse it can lead to a whole range of emotional and psychological problems that are increasingly being treated by psychoanalysis.

Guggul is used to treat lipid disorders.

RIGHT *As well as curing illness, rejuvenation therapy can bring renewed vitality to every aspect of mind and body.*

❖ **Acara rasayana** (for rejuvenation without medicines)

Rejuvenating effects can also be achieved when you practice good conduct, or sadacara. Sadacara includes worship of gods; respect for seniors and elders; avoidance of anger, jealousy, envious and unkind behavior; balanced sleep; regular intake of milk, ghee and other nutritious food; nonsuppression of natural urges; and regular practice of meditation. Good conduct helps to free you from stress and emotional disturbances that are the cause of so many ailments. This makes acara rasayana an ideal therapy for today's fast and stress-filled world.

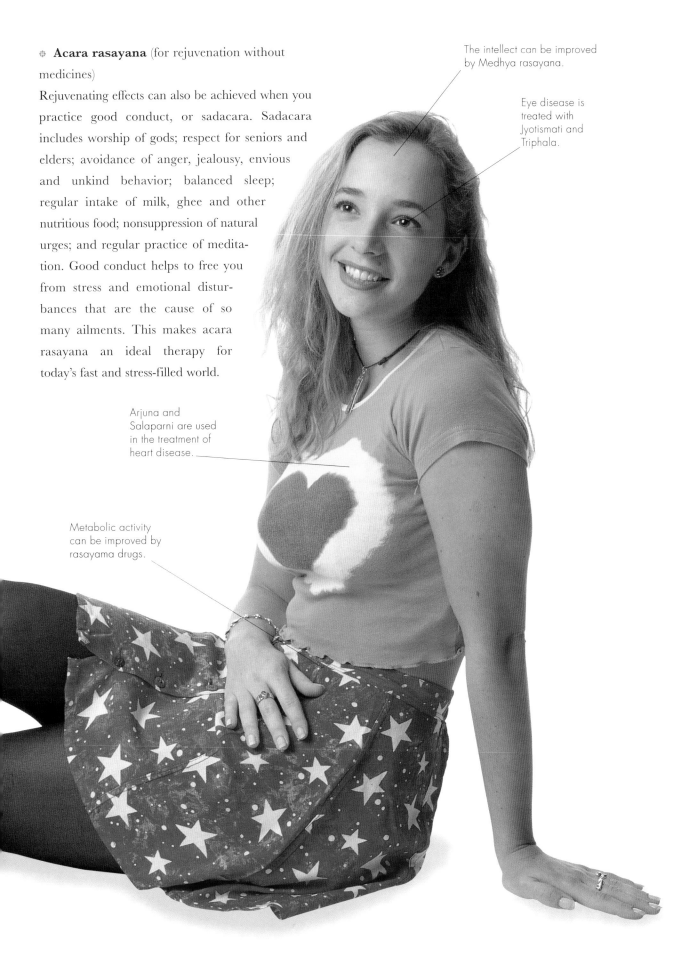

The intellect can be improved by Medhya rasayana.

Eye disease is treated with Jyotismati and Triphala.

Arjuna and Salaparni are used in the treatment of heart disease.

Metabolic activity can be improved by rasayama drugs.

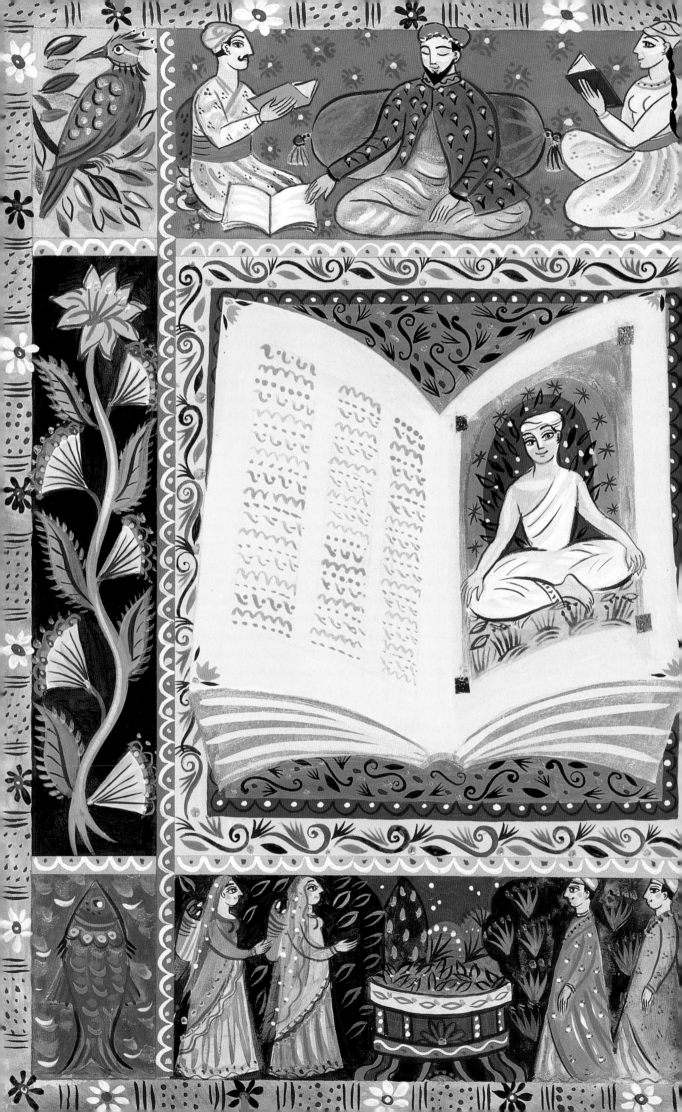

Further Information

}•{

THIS SECTION *of the book provides further information on Ayurveda. A list of useful addresses gives you access to reputable practitioners and suppliers of medicines in different parts of the world. The meanings of the more difficult terms used in this book are fully explained in the glossary which also includes a guide to the pronunciation of many of the Hindu terms used in the book. A further reading list is offered to help readers expand their understanding of Indian philosophy and medicine. An index to all aspects of Ayurvedic medicine is provided at the end of the book.*

Useful Addresses

AYURVEDA COLLEGE

A fully-fledged college of Ayurveda will begin to function from Autumn 1997 in London, in a joint venture between the Ayurvedic Company of Great Britain and the Thames Valley University, and the Wolfson College of Health Science.

This college will offer a four-year full-time university degree course in Ayurveda for school leavers with requisite A-levels as well as a part-time program for nurses, medical physicians, and graduate professionals.

Faculty for the course will consist of Ayurvedic physicians from India and Europe.

Those seeking admission may write to :
Ayurvedic Company of Great Britain
50 Penywern Road
London, SW5 9SX
United Kingdom

AYURVEDA COLLEGES

College of Ayurveda
Arya Vaidya Pharmacy
1382 Trichy Road
Coimbatore 641018
South India

College of Ayurveda
Arya Vaidya Sala Hospital
Kottakkal 676503
Dist: Mallapuram
Kerala State
South India

College of Ayurveda
Ayurvedic Company of
Great Britain
50 Penywern Road
London, SW5 9SX
United Kingdom

Faculty of Ayurveda
Institute of Medical Sciences
Benaras Hindu University
Varanasi - 221005
India

AYURVEDIC & HERBAL INSTITUTIONS IN THE WEST

**American Institute
of Vedic Studies**
PO Box 8357
Santa Fe, NM 87504
U.S.A.

**The Ayurvedic Institute
of Wellness Centre**
1131 Menual N.E., Suite
Albuquerque, NM 87112
U.S.A.

Maharishi Ayurveda
579 Punt Road
South Yarra
Victoria 3141
Australia

The Ayurvedic Institute
PO Box 282
Fairfield
Iowa, 52556
U.S.A.

AYURVEDIC HOSPITALS IN INDIA

Arya Vaidya Pharmacy
1382 Trichy Road
Coimbatore 641018
South India

Arya Vaidya Sala Hospital
Kottakkal 676503
Dist: Mallapuram
Kerala State
South India

ASSOCIATIONS

**Council for Complementary
and Alternative Medicine**
19a Cavendish Square
London, W1M 9AD
United Kingdom

**Maharishi Ayur-Veda
Health Centre**
24 Linhope Street,
London, NW1 6HT
United Kingdom

**North African Centre
of Medicinal Plants**
Pharmacognosy Department
Faculty of Pharmacy
University of Cairo
Kasr. El. Aini.
Egypt

**Academie International
des Medecines Naturelles**
52 boulevard Flandrin
75116 Paris
France

**Syndicat National
des Producteurs,
Ramasseurs et Collecteurs
de Plantes
Medicinales, Aromatiques
et Industrielles**
6 blvd Joffre,
91490 Milly
France

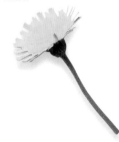

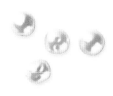

**Japan Institute of
Traditional Medicine**
Chushoto Building
3–4–10 Nihonbashi
Chio-ku
Tokyo 103
Japan

**Research Institute for
Wakan-Yaku**
Toyama Medical and
Pharmaceutical University
2630 Suyitami
Toyama-shi 930–01
Japan

**Instituto Mexicano
de Seguro Social**
Unidad de Investigacion en
Medicina
Tradicional y Desarrolo de
Medicamentos
Calle Argentina 1
C P 62790 Xochitepec Morales
Mexico

Economic Botany Symposium
New York Botanical Gardens
Bronx, New York 10458
U.S.A.

**American Association of
Ayurvedic Medicine**
P.O. Box 598
South Lancaster
Massachusetts 01561
U.S.A.

**American Holistic Medical
Association**
4101 Lake Boone Trail,
Suite 201,
Raleigh,
North Carolina 27607
U.S.A.

Herbal Gram
PO Box 12006
Austin
Texas 78711
U.S.A.

**Napralert (Natural
Product Database)**
The University of Illinois
Box 6998, Chicago
Illinois 60680
U.S.A.

AYURVEDIC
PRODUCTS SUPPLIERS

**Ayurvedic Company of
Great Britain Limited**
50 Penywern Road
London, SW5 9SX
United Kingdom

Arya Vaidya Pharmacy
1382 Trichy Road
Coimbatore 641018
South India

Arya Vaidya Sala Hospital
Kottakkal 676503
Dist: Mallapuram
Kerala State
South India

Ajanta Pharma Limited
98 Govt. Industrial Area
Charkop, Kandivili (W)
Mumbai 400 067
India

Ayurved Vikas Sansthan
C-83 Gandhi Nagar
Moradabad 244001
India

**Shree Baidyanath Ayurved
Bhawan Ltd**
1 Gupta Lane
Calcutta 700 006
India

Cholayil Pharmaceuticals
No 4 M-Block
Anna Nagar East
Madras 600 102
India

Dabur India Limited
22 Site IV, Sahibabad
Ghaziabad 201 010
India

**Deshrakshak Aushdhalaya
Limited**
Kankhal 249408
Haridwar (UP)
India

**Shree Dhootapapeshwar
Limited**
135 Nanubhai Desai Road
Khetwadi, Mumbai 400 004
India

Kerala Ayurveda Pharmacy Ltd
PO No. 2, Aluva,
Kerala 683 101
South India

Lupin Laboraties Limited
159 C. S. T. Road
Kalina
Santacruz (East)
Bombay 400 098
India

Unique
'Neelam Centre' 'B' Wing,
4th Floor, Hind Cycle Road,
Worli, Bombay 400 025
India

Zandu
70 Gokhale Road (South)
Dadar, Bombay 400 025
India

Aphrodesia Products, Inc.
264 Bleeker Street,
New York 10014
U.S.A.

Glossary

A guide to pronunciation is given for each entry in the Glossary. Capitals indicate which syllables should be stressed.

Agni (UG-ni) – Agni literally means "fire," but when used in Ayurveda implies the various factors that take part in the digestion and metabolism of food at all levels.

Ahara (ah-HAH-ra) – This means diet. Any impairment of nutrition as a result of unwholesome ahara, or diet, results in diseases. Thus ahara is an important aspect of treatment.

Ahita (a-HIT-a) – That which is not good or wholesome for life is Ahita.

Akasha (ah-KAH-sha) – One of the panchamahabhutas – the five eternal substances responsible for the creation of all material substances in this universe.

Ama (AH-ma) – Relates to the state of food ingested as a result of impaired functioning of the agni. In other words, uncooked, immature, or undigested food is ama.

Antah pari marjana (un-tukh-purr-i-MURR-ja-na) – The method of treatment where internal purification is done not only with the help of different types of drugs but also special purificatory measures known as panchakarma.

Artha (URR-ta) – In the present context, the word means wealth or riches.

Asana (AH-sa-na) – Term given to various yogic postures that form an important aspect of the practice of yoga. Literally, the term means "making oneself sit in a comfortable position."

Asatmyendriyartha samyoga (a-saht-myenn-DREE-ya-urr-ta-sum-YO) – This refers to the unwholesome or stressful contact of the sense organs with other objects, thereby causing the excitement of the doshas (the three basic factors).

Astavidha pariksha (a-shtah-vid-a-pa-REEK-shah) – The term for the eightfold general examination of the patient. This includes the examination of nadi (pulse), jivha (tongue), sabda (voice), trak (skin), drka (vision), akrti (general appearance), mutra (urine), and mala (stool).

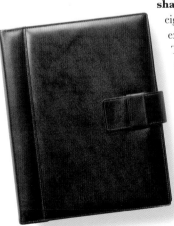

Bheda (BHAY-da) – This is the last stage of kriyakala when the disease may become chronic and cause complications.

Bhuta (BHOO-ta) – The five eternal substances or panchamahabhutas are singularly referred to as bhuta.

Brahma (brukh-MAH) – The Hindu god known as the creator of the universe, and the original propounder of Ayurveda.

Charaka (CHURR-a-ka) – Charaka is the physician who propagated his knowledge of medicine and is the author of the text *Charaka samhita*.

Dhanwantari (dhunn-VUNN-ta-ri) – Surgeon of gods.

Dharma (DHURR-ma) – The correct duty or action for your life.

Dhatus (DHAH-toos) – These are the units of the body tissues and are seven in number. They are rasa, rakta, mamsa, meda, asthi, majja, and shukra.

Dinacharya (dinn-a-churr-YAH) – The daily routine that includes all aspects of regimen and diet, to stay healthy and happy.

Dosha (DOH-sha) – The three basic elements of the body – vata, pitta, and kapha. These are responsible for the entire physiological phenomena in our body.

Dukha (DOOKH-a) – This means misery or unhappiness, as a result of sinful acts.

Durga (door-GAH) – Hindu goddess and an incarnation of Parvati, the wife of Shiva.

Ganapathy (gunn-a-PUTT-i) – The elephant-headed Hindu god and son of Shiva and Parvati.

Grishma (greesh-MAH) – Summer.

Guggul (GOOG-ool-a) – An exudate from the bark of Commiphora mukul, used as medicine in Ayurveda.

Guna (GOON-a) – This refers to a property of a substance, whether physical, chemical or pharmacological

Hemanta (hay-MAHN-ta) – Early winter.

Hita (HIT-a) – This refers to an advantageous or good or useful state.

Jala (JULL-a) – One of the five basic elements (mahabhutas), jala is water.

Kali (KAH-lee) – Hindu goddess and an incarnation of Parvati.

Kama (KAH-ma) – Gratification or fulfilment of desire.

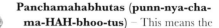

Kapha (KUFF-a) – This is one of the three doshas. Kapha takes part in all constructive activities of our system and has a heavy, viscous, slimy, stable, and sturdy form.

Kriyakala (kree-yah-KAH-la) – This is defined as the stage or stages in the process of a disease that gives ample opportunity to understand the disease and to resort to therapeutic measures. There are six stages of kriyakala – sanchaya, prakopa, prasara, sthavasamraya, vyakti, and bheda.

Mahabharata (ma-hah-BHAH-ra-ta) – The great Indian epic, full of moral values and great teachings.

Malas (MULL-a(s)) – The malas in Ayurveda represent a wide variety of substances but in a wider sense it means waste products or excretions. The feces, urine, sweat, bile, excretions of ear, skin, and nose are all included in malas.

Mantra (MUNN-tra) – A mystical syllable, word, or phrase used to focus the mind during meditation. Om is the best known mantra.

Maya (mah-YAH) – Illusion used primarily to describe the relative nature of human reality.

Moksha (MOKK-sha) – The liberation from worldly desires or final emanicaption is moksha.

Nadi (NAH-dee) – The pulse is referred to as nadi in Ayurveda. This is a part of the astavidha pariksha, the eightfold clinical examination of the patient.

Nasya (NUSS-ya) – This is a type of panchakarma procedure (purification measure) where medicines, whether liquids or powders or oils, are given through the nose to get the desired response.

Nidana (ni-DAH-na) – In Ayurveda, this refers to the etiological factors or causative factors of the diseases. These causative factors or nidanas are indicative of the disease that may arise in future.

Panchakarma (punn-nya-cha-KAHR-ma) – This is a fivefold purification therapy and is a classical form of treatment in Ayurveda. These specialized procedures include emesis, purgation, enema (decoction and oily), and nasal insufflation.

Panchamahabhutas (punn-nya-cha-ma-HAH-bhoo-tus) – This means the five basic eternal substances – akasha (space), vayu (air), agni (fire), jala (water), and prthvi (earth). The Ayurveda theory of creation believes these five eternal substances to be responsible for the creation of all living beings. These are the ultimate substances from which the material world is derived.

Parinama (purr-i-NAH-ma) – In common parlance, this means the result. Ayurveda believes that as a result of seasonal changes, specifically marked with traits that are contrary to its true nature, a number of diseases may arise. So, this Parinama has been included in the etiology of the diseases along with the other causative factors.

Parvati (pahr-va-TEE) – Hindu goddess and wife of Shiva.

Pitta (PITT-a) – One of the three doshas. Pitta is responsible for all biochemical activities and is represented by its main property, heat, besides the other attributes.

Prajnaparadha (prujj-nyah-pa-RAH-dha) – This is the term used for an impaired intellect and memory, which ultimately results in the development of an illness, whether physical or mental.

Prakopa (pra-KOH-pa) – The three doshas, or basic units, get excited due to exposure to various etiological factors, after the first stage of accumulation or sanchaya. This excitation is given the terminology of prakopa.

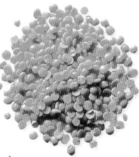

Prakriti (PRUKK-er-ti) – Prakriti is also used as the feminine aspect of creation as opposed to purusha, the male principle.

Prakrti (PRUKK-er-ti) – The human constitution has been given a psychosomatic entity in Ayurveda, and the term prakrti is used for defining the same. This prakrti has been discussed in relevance to the tridoshas, and based on the relative preponderance of each, the constitution has been divided into seven categories – vataja, pittaja, kaphaja, vata pittaja, vata kaphaja, pitta kaphaja, and samdoshaja.

Glossary

Prashama (pra-SHUMM-a) – The term literally means remission. The doshas, after their accumulation of excitation, may pass to the stage of prashama (remission) and not proceed to further stages of disease, if the exciting factors are not strong enough.

Prthvi (per-TVEE) – The term is used for earth, which forms one of the five basic eternal substances (panchamahabhutas).

Purusha (POOR-oosh-a) – An individual being or self. A male principle in the creation of the universe.

Purvaroopa (poohr-va-ROO-pa) – The premonitory symptoms of a disease, before it is fully manifested are known as purvaroopa. The purvaroopa helps not only to understand the disease at its early stage, and the course it would take, but also to plan the therapy.

Rajas (RUJJ-us) – One of the properties of the psyche or mind and the most active and responsible for different motions.

Rasayana (ra-SHA-ya-na) – The rasayana is the rejuvenation therapy and forms one of the eight clinical specialties of Ayurveda. The therapy aims at promotion of strength and vitality, and imparts immunity against diseases thus increasing your longevity.

Rig Veda (rig-VAY-da) – This is one of the four *Vedas* – the divine books of knowledge of the Hindus.

Ritucharya (rit-ooch-urr-YAH) – This refers to the seasonal regimen. For every season a different regimen has been prescribed to enable a person to lead a healthy life by overcoming the stresses brought on by the seasonal changes.

Roopa (ROO-pa) – This term carries two meanings in Ayurveda – (1) shape or color and (2) signs and symptoms of a disease. The second holds great importance and it is directly related to diagnosis and treatment.

Samprapti (sum-PRAHP-ti) – The complete phenomena from the aggravation of the doshas to the complete manifestation of a disease is samprapti. Thus, in a broader sense, the term indicates the pathogenesis of a disease.

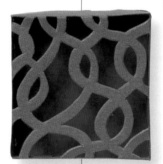

Sanchaya (summ-SAH-ra) – This is the first stage of kriyakala (the process of manifestation of a disease). The stage represents the start of the disease, with the accumulation, or sanchaya, of the doshas in their own sites in our body.

Sastra pranidhana (shuss-tra-prunn-i-DHAH-na) – This means surgical treatment.

Sattva (SUTT-va) – One of the properties of the mind or psyche and characterized by clarity of mind, harmony of the senses, and the proper perception of knowledge. Also a term used for mana, or mind.

Satwavajaya (sutt-vah-va-JY-a) – This is a method of treatment in mental disorders (psychotherapy). The therapy aims at controlling the mind away from the unwholesome desires. This is best achieved by concentration, spiritual knowledge, understanding, and control of mind or will.

Shakti (SHUKK-ti) – The female energy that dominates prakrti, the manifested universe.

Shiva (SHIV-a) – Hindu god of destruction and creation and auspiciousness.

Sisira (shi-SHIR-a) – Late winter.

Snehana (snay-HANN-a) – Oil therapy used to prepare the body for treatment. May be administered through different kinds of food or by enema or massage.

Sthana samsraya (stah-na-sum-SHRY-a) – This is the fourth stage of kriyakala, where the doshas, after their accumulation, aggravation, and spread get localized in the particular tissue or organ. The localization is termed as sthanasamsraya, and it occurs in weakened organs or tissues.

Sukha (SOOKH-a) – Happiness and harmony.

Sushruta (soosh-ROOT-a) – He is the author of *Sushruta samhita* – a text book on surgery. He is also known as the father of ancient Indian surgery.

Swedana (SVAY-da-na) – Fomentation therapy given to patients after massage or snehana, to prepare the patient for the main panchakarma treatment. Swedana is done in a wide variety of ways depending upon the disease, the condition of the doshas, and the patient.

Tamas (TAM-us) – The property of the mind or psyche or manas and characterized by inertia, inactivity, and disturbed perception and activities of the mind.

Tejas (TAY-jus) – One of the bhutas forming a part of the panchamahabhuta and having the characteristics of fire. The pitta dosha is formed by the predominance of tejamahabhuta.

Tridoshas (tri-DOH-sha(s)) – The three basic fundamental units in a human body – vata, pitta, and kapha. These three doshas govern the entire physiological phenomena in a living being, with their respective functional activities.

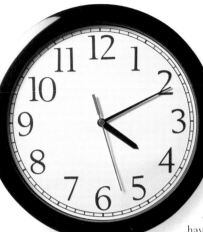

Upasaya (oop-a-SHY-a) – This is the exploratory therapy, generally done for a differential diagnosis, when it is difficult to differentiate and arrive at a diagnosis. This is achieved through factors such as medicine, diet, and regimen.

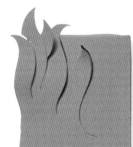

Vahirparimarjana (vah-hir-purr-i-MURR-ja-na) – This refers to the external treatment measures such as oleation, fomentation, baths, application of pastes and powders, and medicated gargles. These measures can be used along with internal medicine or even independently, depending upon the disease and the type of therapy planned.

Vajikarana (vah-jee-KURR-a-na) – The type of therapy that aims at improving the virility of a man is known as Vajikarana. These agents are a separate class of drugs and the main object is fulfilment of the desire to produce progeny by improving the virility.

Vamana (VUMM-a-na) – Emesis therapy, administered to eliminate waste products through the upper pathway (mouth) by way of vomiting. This is part of panchakarma treatment (fivefold therapeutic procedures). The vamana treatment is specifically used when the kapha dosha is the dominant one in the pathogenesis of a disease.

Varsha (vurr-SHAH) – Rains (rainy season).

Vasanta (va-SUNN-ta) – Spring.

Vata (VAH-ta) – One of the tridoshas, and responsible for all motions and actions.

Vayu (vah-YOO) – Synonym for vata.

Vedas (VAY-da(s)) – The divine books of knowledge of Hindus compiled during the period 1500 to 800 BC. There are four *Vedas* – *Rig Veda, Sama Veda, Atharva Veda* and *Yajur Veda,* each dealing with various aspects of Indian culture, philosophy, and healing art.

Vihara (vi-HAH-ra) – Mode of living or lifestyle is vihara. In Ayurveda strict rules regarding vihara have been laid down as regards the diseases, seasons, and daily routine in a healthy and diseased individual.

Virecana (vi-RAY-cha-na) – The purgation therapy is virecana and is a part of the panchakarma therapy. This is usually administered where pitta dosha is predominant and therefore responsible for the disease.

Vishnu (VISH-noo) – Hindu god responsible for preservation of the world. Dhanwantari, the god of Ayurveda is considered an incarnation of Vishnu.

Vyakti (VYUKK-ti) – The fifth stage of kriyakala (process of manifestation of disease) where the disease becomes fully manifested with all its signs and symptoms.

Yoga (YOH-ga) – To unite or to integrate, i.e. the union of individual soul with the supreme soul. In the ultimate sense, this system helps in the physical, mental, and spiritual development.

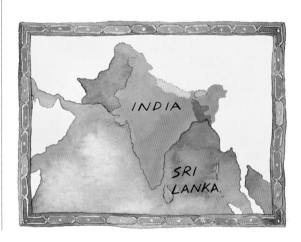

Further Reading

Health Essentials: Ayurveda – The Ancient Indian Healing Art. Scott Gerson M.D. Element, 1993.

The Bhagavad Gita – Any edition.

Caraka Samhita. P.V. Sharma, Delhi, London: Chaukhambha Orietalia, 1981.

Sushrata Samhita. Translated by K.L. Bhishagratna (Sanskrit series). Varanasi, India: Chaukhambha, 1981.

Indian Materia Medica: Volumes One and Two. Dr. K. M. Madkarni.

The Yoga of Herbs: An Ayurvedic Guide to Herbal Medicine. Dr. David Frawley and Dr. Vasant Lad. Sate Fe: Lotus Press, 1988.

Prakrti: Your Ayurvedic Constitution. Robert E. Svoboda. Albuquerque: Geocom Press, 1988.

Madhava Nidanam (Roga Viniscaya) of Madhavakara: A Treatise on Ayurveda. Jaikrishnadas Ayurveda Series, 69. Prof. K. R., Srikanta Murthy. New Delhi, India: Chaukhambha Orientalia, 1987.

A Handbook of Ayurveda. Vaidya Bhagwan Dash and Acarya Manfred M. Junius. New Delhi, India: Concept Publishing Co., 1983.

Doctrines of Pathology in Ayurveda. Vidyavilas Ayurveda Series, 3. Prof. K. R. Srikantha Murthy, Varansani, India: Chaukhambha Prietalia, 1987.

Basic Principles of Ayurveda. Bhagwan Dash. New Delhi, India: Concept Publishing Co., 1980.

Ayurvedic Medicine, Past and Present. Pandit Shiv Sharma. Calcutta, India: Dabur Publications, 1975.

The Potential for Herbal Medicines in the World Pharmaceutical Industry. McAlpine, Thorpe & Warrier Limited, 1988.

Future World Trends in the Supply, Utilisation and Marketing of Endangered Medicinal Plants. McAlpine, Thorpe & Warrier Limited, 1995.

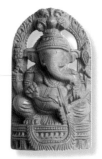

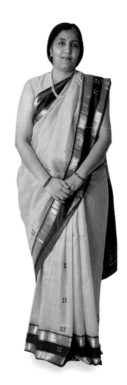

Who's Who in the World Herbal Medical Industry. McAlpine, Thorpe & Warrier Limited, 1995.

Hindu Goddesses: Visions of the Divine Feminine in the Hindu Religious Tradition. David Kinsley. Motilal Banarsidass.

The Divine Player. David Kinsley. Motilal Banarsidass.

An Advanced History of India. Majumdar, R.C., H.C. Rachaudhuri, and Kalikinkar Datta. New York: St. Martin's Press, 1967.

The Siva-Purana. Translated by a Board of Scholars. 4 vols. Delhi: Motilal Banarsidass, 1970.

Nataraja in Art, Thought and Literature. New Delhi: National Museum, 1974.

Taittiriya-aranyaka. 3d ed. 2 vols. Poona: Anandasrama Sanskrit Series, 1967-69.

Taittiriya-brahmana. 2 vols. Poona: Anandasrama Sanskrit Series, 1934, 1938.

The Vishnu purana, a System of Hindu Mythology and Tradition. Translated by H.H. Wilson. 3d ed. Calcutta: Punthi Pustak, 1961.

Index